AYURVEDA
The Science of Self~Healing
by Dr. Vasant Lad

A PRACTICAL GUIDE

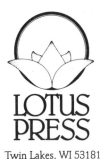

LOTUS PRESS

Twin Lakes, WI 53181

This book is a reference work based on the author's educational teaching and practical experience. The information contained herein is in no way to be considered as a substitute for consultation with a duly licensed physician.

REPRINTED 2009
PUBLISHED IN 2004 BY:
LOTUS PRESS
P.O. Box 325 Twin Lakes, WI 53181 USA
Phone: (262) 889-8561 Fax: (262) 889-2461
(email) lotuspress@lotuspress.com (website) www.lotuspress.com

Excerpt from WHO DIES by Stephan Levine. Copyright © 1982 by Stephan Levine. Reprinted by permission of Doubleday & Company, Inc.

SECOND EDITION, 1985
Printed in the United States of America

Library of Congress Cataloging in Publication Data
Lad, Vasant, 1943-
    Ayurveda: the science of self-healing

    Bibliography: p. 171
    Includes index.
    1. Medicine, Ayurvedic. 2. Health. 1. Title
R605 L26   1984   610   83-80620
ISBN: 978-0-9149-5500-9

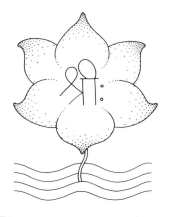

Dedicated to Mother, Father,
Satguru-Hambir Baba and Dear Pappu,
who taught me about life, love, compassion,
simplicity and humility.

श्री दि
Kashi ॐ

Acknowledgements

This author wishes to acknowledge the following individuals whose efforts have contributed to the creation of the text:

Angela Werneke, artist, who is responsible for all the art contained in this book including the cover, charts, diagrams and tables. Angela's work has contributed an additional dimension to the book.

David Mackenzie, photographer, whose overall input on the artistic presentation is much appreciated.

Malinda Elliott and **Harriet Slavitz,** editors, who spent much time and effort and gave their total dedication in preparing the manuscript.

Lavon Alt, typist, who produced the index.

Susan Voorhees, Becky Vogel, Peter Fisk and **Win Hampton,** models, who gave their time and effort in posing for the photographs.

Jim Redlich, for his support and commitment to Ayurveda.

Lenny Blank. Lastly, the author wishes to express here a special thanks to Lennyji, who has provided the guidance and inspiration for the book. Without his total commitment and dedication, this book would still be lying on the shelf of this author's mind. There are no words to express this person's gratitude to my dearest friend.

TABLE OF CONTENTS

Preface 13
Chapter I - History and Philosophy 15
    A. The First Life Science 18
    B. Ayurveda and Human Potential 18
    C. Ayurveda, Yoga and Tantra 18
    D. Ayurveda and The Western Mind 19
Chapter II - The Five Elements and Man 21
    A. Man as Microcosm 22
    B. The Senses 23
Chapter III - The Human Constitution 26
    A. Understanding Tridosha 29
    B. Determining the Individual Constitution 31
    C. Vata Constitution 31
    D. Pitta Constitution 32
    E. Kapha Constitution 33
    F. Mental Constitutions 36
Chapter IV - Disease Process 37
    A. Disease Classification 37
    B. Disease Proneness 38
    C. Key to Health or Disease — 'Agni' 39
    D. Repressed Emotions 40
    E. The Three Malas 41
    F. The Seven Dhatus 44
Chapter V - Attributes 48
Chapter VI - Diagnosis 52
    A. Examination of the Radial Pulse 52
    B. Tongue Diagnosis 59
    C. Facial Diagnosis 62
    D. Lip Diagnosis 64
    E. Nail Diagnosis 64
    F. Eye Diagnosis 67

Chapter VII - Treatment 69
   A. Emotional Release 69
   B. The Pancha Karma 70
      1. Therapeutic Vomiting (*Vaman*) 70
      2. Purgatives (*Virechan*) 70
      3. Enema (*Basti*) 73
      4. Nasal Administration (*Nasya*) 75
      5. Blood-Letting (*Rakta Moksha*) 78
   C. Palliation 79
Chapter VIII - Diet 80
   A. Fasting 85
   B. Vitamins 87
Chapter IX - Taste 88
   A. Rasa, Virya and Vipak 88
Chapter X - Lifestyle and Routine 100
   A. Suggestions for a Creative, Healthy Life 101
      1. Routine 101
      2. Diet and Digestion 101
      3. Physical Hygiene 102
      4. Mental Hygiene 103
Chapter XI - Time 104
   A. Sun and Moon 105
   B. Astrology 107
   C. Ages of Human Life 107
Chapter XII - Longevity 109
   A. Yoga 113
   B. Breathing and Meditation (*Pranayama*) 114
   C. Mantra 125
   D. Meditation 125
   E. Massage 128
Chapter XIII - Medicinals 129
   A. The Kitchen Pharmacy 129
   B. Metals 141
   C. Gems, Stones and Color Therapy 144
      1. Calendar of Birth Stones 145
      2. Uses of Gems 145
   D. Color 148

Conclusion 151
Appendices
   Appendix A - Food Antidotes 154
   Appendix B - First Aid Treatments 157
   Appendix C - Recipes 162
Glossary 164
Bibliography 171
Index 172

List of Tables, Charts & Diagrams

Table 1 — The Five Elements, the Organs of the Senses and
　　　　　 Their Actions 24
Table 2 — The Human Constitution (Prakruti) 34
Table 3 — The Twenty Attributes (Gunas) and Their Actions . . . 50
Table 4 — Attributes of the Tri-dosha 51
Table 5 — Food Guidelines for Basic Constitutional Types 82
Table 6 — Tastes and Their Actions 90
Table 7 — Properties and Actions of Rasa, Virya, Vipak 92
Table 8 — Asanas for Derangement of Vata, Pitta, Kapha 123

Chart　1 — Samkhya Philosophy of Creation 17
Chart　2 — Functions of Tri-dosha 28
Chart　3 — Examination of Urine 43
Chart　4 — The Circulation of Nutrients and
　　　　　　 Transformation of Dhatus 46
Chart　5 — Emesis Therapy (Vaman) 71
Chart　6 — Purgation Therapy (Virechan) 72
Chart　7 — Enema Therapy (Basti) 74
Chart　8 — Nasal Administration (Nasya) 76
Chart　9 — Tri-Dosha Mandala 106
Chart 10 — Yoga Postures for Vata, Pitta, Kapha Ailments 115

Diagram　1 — The Seats of Vata, Pitta, Kapha 27
Diagram　2 — (Nadi) Pulse Diagnosis 53
Diagram 2A — Identification of the Pulse 54
Diagram　3 — Pulse Points 55
Diagram　4 — The Meridians and
　　　　　　　　 The Basic Five Elements 57
Diagram　5 — The Pulse and The Organs 58
Diagram　6 — Tongue Diagnosis (Jihva) 60
Diagram　7 — Facial Diagnosis 63
Diagram　8 — Lip Diagnosis (Ostha) 65
Diagram　9 — Nail Diagnosis 66
Diagram 10 — Eye Diagnosis 67
Diagram 11 — So-Hum Meditation 127

PREFACE

The author's inspiration for this book grew out of a strong belief that Ayurveda should be shared with Westerners in a simple, practical way. Heretofore, Ayurveda has been viewed in the West as an esoteric science. Yet it is a simple, practical science of life whose principles are universally applicable to each individual's daily existence. Ayurveda speaks to every element and facet of human life, offering guidance that has been tested and refined over many centuries to all those who seek greater harmony and peace and longevity.

The knowledge supplied in this book will be of lasting value to the reader. The science of Ayurveda is based not on constantly changing research data, but on the eternal wisdom of the *rishis* who received this science, expressive of the perfect wholeness of Cosmic Consciousness, through religious introspection and meditation. Ayurveda is a timeless science and the reflection and elucidation here, it is hoped, will serve the reader throughout his or her life.

Ayurveda is concerned with eight principle branches of medicine: pediatrics, gynecology, obstetrics, ophthalmology, geriatrics, otolaryngology (ear, nose and throat), general medicine and surgery. Each of these medical specialties is addressed according to theories of the five elements (Ether, Air, Fire, Water, Earth); the *tridosha*, or three bodily humors; the seven *dhatus*, or body tissues; three *malas* (urine, stools, sweat); and the trinity of life: body, mind and spiritual awareness. These concepts are fully elucidated in this introductory text.

This book is mainly concerned with presenting a basic overview of Ayurveda, including techniques of examination, diagnosis and treatment; promotion of longevity; the use of herbal remedies and other practical everyday aspects of maintaining health.

Once the student has acquired a basic overview of Ayurveda, a wealth of ancient knowledge still remains to be explored in writings of the Ayurvedic sages, such as the surgeon Sushruta (who, more than 2,000 years ago, wrote a classic text on surgery, *Sushruta Samhita*), and through the teachings of modern Ayurvedic physicians. The writings of Sushruta impressively anticipated much of modern medicine. He treated in detail, among other topics, postmortem dissection and plastic surgery procedures which, centuries later, were used as the basis for modern plastic surgery. Sushruta perfected techniques for knitting broken bones with nails; he identified vital points on the body, *marmas*, which are related to the vital organs. External trauma to these points may be extremely serious or fatal. Among his other numerous contributions, Sushruta also devised a special treatment of bloodletting to cure blood-born disorders. It should be obvious, from this brief highlighting, that we have much to learn from the ancient Ayurvedic masters.

The wisdom of Ayurveda is recorded in Sanskrit, the ancient language of India. Therefore, the author sometimes employs Sanskrit terms to explain certain Ayurvedic medical concepts when no adequate English translation may be made. On their first appearance in this text, each of these words is clearly and simply elucidated.

This is the author's first book, and he wishes to acknowledge his mentors in Ayurveda, especially: Vaidya B.P. Nanal; the Tilak Ayurveda Mahavidhyalaya Medical School where the author studied and was later appointed as a lecturer and professor of Internal Medicine; and the Seth Tarachand Ramnath Ayurvedic Hospital where the author received his practical training as physician in residence and where he later served as Medical Director. In addition he wishes to thank his students and friends whose love, compassion and support inspired him to write this text. He offers thanks also to the reader who, in his commitment to learning and to his own growth process, opens himself to the science of Ayurveda as it is set forth in these pages.

Dr. Vasant Lad
Santa Fe, New Mexico
January 1984

Chapter I
History and Philosophy *

Ayurveda encompasses not only science but religion and philosophy as well. We use the word *religion* to denote beliefs and disciplines conducive toward states of being in which the doors of perception open to all aspects of life. In Ayurveda, the whole of life's journey is considered to be sacred. The word *philosophy* refers to love of truth and in Ayurveda, truth is Being, Pure Existence, The Source of all life. Ayurveda is a science of truth as it is expressed in life.

All Ayurvedic literature is based on the *Samkhya* philosophy of creation. (The roots of the term *Samkhya* are two Sanskrit words: *sat*, meaning "truth," and *khya*, meaning "to know.") The reader is asked to cultivate an open mind and heart toward the philosophy of *Samkhya* because of its intimate connection with Ayurveda.

The ancient realized beings, *rishis*, or seers of truth, discovered truth by means of religious practices and disciplines. Through intensive meditation, they manifested truth in their daily lives. Ayurveda is the science of daily living and this system of knowledge evolved from the *rishis'* practical, philosophical and religious illumination, which was rooted in their understanding of the creation.

They perceived, in the close relationship between man and the universe, how cosmic energy manifests in all living and nonliving things. They also realized that the source of all existence is Cosmic Consciousness, which manifests as male and female energy — *Shiva* and *Shakti*.

The *rishi* Kapila, who realized the *Samkhya* philosophy of creation, discovered twenty-four principles or elements of the universe.**

---

* This chapter, which may be difficult for readers who have no prior knowledge of the subjects discussed, may be read first, last or at any point that is comfortable.

** The specific 24 principles or elements in the Samkhya philosophy are the following: Prakruti; Mahad, Ahamkar; Five Sense Faculties; Five Motor Organs; Mind; Five Senses, i.e.,

15

of which *Prakruti*, or creativity, is the most basic.

Purusha is the male, while *Prakruti* is the female energy. *Purusha* is formless, colorless and beyond attributes and takes no active part in the manifestation of the universe. This energy is choiceless, passive awareness.

Prakruti has form, color and attributes: it is awareness with choice. It is Divine Will, the One who desires to become many. The universe is the child born out of the womb of *Prakruti*, the Divine Mother.

Prakruti creates all forms in the universe, while *Purusha* is the witness to this creation. It is primordial physical energy containing the three attributes, or *gunas*, found in all nature, the evolving cosmos.

The three *gunas* are *satva* (essence), *rajas* (movement) and *tamas* (inertia). These three are the foundation for all existence. They are contained in balance in *Prakruti*. When this balance is disturbed, there is an interaction of the *gunas* which thus engenders the evolution of the universe.

The first manifestation from *Prakruti* is Cosmic Intellect. From *Mahad*, Ego (*Ahamkar*) is formed. Ego then manifests into the five senses (*tanmatras*) and the five motor organs, with the help of *satva*, thus creating the organic universe. The same Ego further manifests into the five basic elements (*bhutas*) with the help of *tamas*, to create the inorganic universe.

Rajas is the active vital life force in the body which moves both the organic and inorganic universes to *satva* and *tamas*, respectively. So *satva* and *tamas* are inactive, potential energies which need the active, kinetic force of *rajas*. *Satva* is creative potential (*Brahma*); *rajas* is a kinetic protective force (*Vishnu*); and *tamas* is a potential destructive force (*Mahesha*). Creation (*Brahma*), Protection (*Vishnu*) and Destruction (*Mahesha*) are the three manifestations of the first cosmic soundless sound, *aum*, which are constantly operating in the universe. The accompanying chart illustrates this manifestation of the universe.

Ether, Air, Fire, Water, Earth. Purusha is often considered to be subsumed under Prakruti, as are the three Gunas, i.e., Satva, Rajas and Tamas. (See Chart 1 on Samkhya Philosophy of Creation.)

16

Chart 1
Samkhya Philosophy of Creation

Purusha is unmanifested, formless, passive, beyond attributes, beyond cause and effect, space and time. *Purusha* is Pure Existence. **Prakruti** is the creative force of action, the source of form, manifestation, attributes and nature. **Mahad** is the Cosmic Intelligence or *Buddhi*. **Ahamkar** is ego, the sense of "I am." **Satva** is stability, pure aspect, awakening, essence and light. **Rajas** is dynamic movement. **Tamas** is static. It is potential energy, inertia, darkness, ignorance and matter.

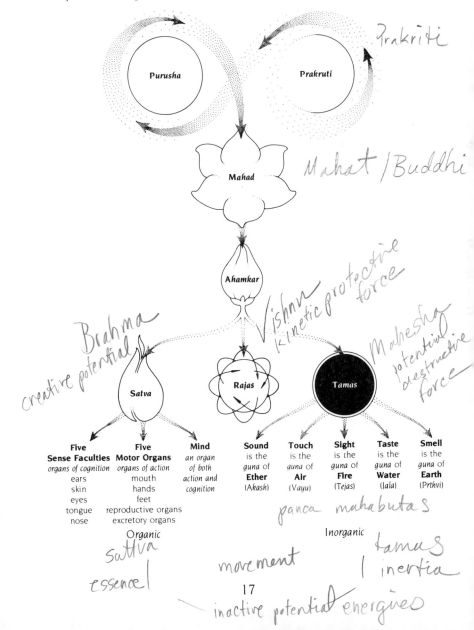

Five Sense Faculties *organs of cognition*	**Five Motor Organs** *organs of action*	**Mind** *an organ of both action and cognition*	**Sound** is the *guna* of **Ether** (Akash)	**Touch** is the *guna* of **Air** (Vayu)	**Sight** is the *guna* of **Fire** (Tejas)	**Taste** is the *guna* of **Water** (Jala)	**Smell** is the *guna* of **Earth** (Prthvi)
ears	mouth						
skin	hands						
eyes	feet						
tongue	reproductive organs						
nose	excretory organs						

Organic

Inorganic

17

THE FIRST LIFE SCIENCE

Ayurveda is a holistic system of medicine that is indigenous to and widely practiced in India. The word Ayurveda is a Sanskrit term meaning "science of life." *Ayu* means "life" or "daily living," and *Veda* is "knowing." Ayurveda was first recorded in the *Vedas*, the world's oldest extant literature. This healing system has been practiced in daily life in India for more than 5,000 years.

AYURVEDA AND HUMAN POTENTIAL

Ayurveda teaches that man is a microcosm, a universe within himself. He is a child of the cosmic forces of the external environment, the macrocosm. His individual existence is indivisible from the total cosmic manifestation. Ayurveda views health and "disease" in holistic terms, taking into consideration the inherent relationship between individual and cosmic spirit, individual and cosmic consciousness, energy and matter.

According to the teachings of Ayurveda, every human being has four biological and spiritual instincts: religious, financial, procreative and the instinct toward freedom. Balanced good health is the foundation for the fulfillment of these instincts. Ayurveda helps the healthy person to maintain health, and the diseased person to regain health. It is a medical-metaphysical healing life-science, the mother of all healing arts. The practice of Ayurveda is designed to promote human happiness, health and creative growth.

Through studying the teachings of Ayurveda, the practical knowledge of self-healing may be acquired by anyone. By the proper balance of all energies in the body, the processes of physical deterioration and disease can be impressively reduced. This concept is basic to Ayurvedic science: the capability of the individual for self-healing.

AYURVEDA, YOGA AND TANTRA

Ayurveda, Yoga and Tantra are the ancient life-disciplines that have been practiced in India for centuries. They are mentioned in the scriptures of the *Vedas* and *Upanishads*. Yoga is the science of union with the Divine, with Truth; Tantra is the most direct method

18

of controlling the energy that creates the ultimate union with Truth; and Ayurveda is the science of life.

The purpose of each practice is to help the individual to achieve longevity, rejuvenation and self-realization. The object of the practices of Yoga and Tantra is liberation, although only certain disciplined individuals are able to achieve this ultimate goal through these practices. However, Ayurveda can be practiced successfully by anyone for the achievement of good health and longevity.

In the spiritual evolution of a man, Ayurveda is the foundation, Yoga is the body and Tantra is the head. It is necessary first to understand Ayurveda in order to experience the practices of Yoga and Tantra. Thus, Ayurveda, Yoga and Tantra form an interdependent trinity of life. None of these practices stands alone. The health of the body, mind* and consciousness** depends on the knowledge and practice of these three in daily life.

AYURVEDA AND THE WESTERN MIND

Western medicine and thinking tend to generalize and to categorize individuality. For instance, according to the Western concept of normality, what is common in a majority of people constitutes the norm. Ayurveda holds that normality must be evaluated individually, because every human constitution manifests its own particular and spontaneous temperament and functioning.

In the East, the key to understanding is acceptance, observation and experience; in the West, it is questioning, analysis and logical deduction. The Western mind, generally, trusts objectivity, while the Eastern gives more emphasis to subjectivity. Eastern science teaches one to go beyond the division between subjectivity and objectivity. This difference in approach may explain why some Westerners experience difficulty in comprehending the methodology of Ayurveda.

Many statements made in this introductory text on Ayurveda

---

* "Mind" in this context, and in the following pages, denotes the operations of the reasoning intellect.
** "Consciousness" here denotes the intuitive operations of the soul in direct communication with the Divine Principle and Source of all life.

19

may elicit the questions, "How?" and "Why?" The author reminds the reader that such questions, though inevitable, are not always answerable. Even in modern Western medicine, some concepts are proven to "work" without the reasons behind the phenomena being fully understood; e.g., though antibiotics are used to destroy the bacteria which form toxins in the body, no adequate explanation exists to explain how and why toxins are formed from bacteria. Furthermore, Ayurveda is truly a holistic science, one in which the sum of many elements comprises its Truth. To question details before a strong overview of the whole science is acquired will prove unproductive and unsatisfactory. The reader is therefore respectfully advised provisionally to accept statements that may at first appear to lack adequate explanation, until he has begun to master the body of Ayurvedic knowledge as a whole.

CHAPTER II

The Five Elements and Man

Ayurveda evolved in the meditative minds of seers of truth, the *rishis*. For thousands of years their teachings were transmitted orally from teacher to disciple, and later they were set down in melodious Sanskrit poetry. Though many of these texts have been lost over time, an abundant body of Ayurvedic knowledge survives.

Originating in Cosmic Consciousness, this wisdom was intuitively received in the hearts of the *rishis*. They perceived that consciousness was energy manifested into the five basic principles, or elements: Ether (space), Air, Fire, Water and Earth. This concept of the five elements lies at the heart of Ayurvedic science.

The *rishis* perceived that in the beginning the world existed in an unmanifested state of consciousness. From that state of unified consciousness, the subtle vibrations of the cosmic soundless sound *aum* manifested. From that vibration there first appeared the Ether element. This ethereal element then began to move; its subtle movements created the Air, which is Ether in action. The movement of Ether produced friction, and through that friction heat was generated. Particles of heat-energy combined to form intense light and from this light the Fire element manifested.

Thus, Ether manifested into Air, and it was the same Ether that further manifested into Fire. Through the heat of the Fire, certain ethereal elements dissolved and liquified, manifesting the Water element, and then solidified to form the molecules of Earth. In this way, Ether manifested into the four elements of Air, Fire, Water and Earth.

From Earth, all organic living bodies, including those in the vegetable kingdom such as herbs and grains, and those in the animal kingdom, including man, are created. Earth also contains the inorganic substances that comprise the mineral kingdom. Thus, out of the womb of the Five Elements all matter is born.

The five basic elements exist in all matter. Water provides the classic example: the solid state of water, ice, is a manifestation of the Earth principle. Latent heat (Fire) in the ice liquifies it, manifesting the Water principle; and then eventually it turns into steam, expressing the Air principle. The steam disappears into Ether, or space. Thus the five basic elements, Ether, Air, Fire, Water and Earth, are present in one substance. All five originated in the energy issuing from Cosmic Consciousness; all five are present in all matter in the universe. Thus, energy and matter are one.

MAN AS MICROCOSM

Man is a microcosm of nature and so the five basic elements present in all matter also exist within each individual. In the human body are many spaces which are manifestations of the Ether element. There are, for example, the spaces in the mouth, nose, gastrointestinal tract, respiratory tract, abdomen, thorax, capillaries, lymphatics, tissues and cells.

Space in movement is called Air. Air is the second cosmic element, the element of movement. Within the human body, Air manifests in the larger movements of the muscles, the pulsations of the heart, the expansion and contraction of the lungs and the movements of the stomach wall and intestines. Under a microscope, even single cells may be seen to move. Response to a stimulus is the movement of afferent and efferent nerve impulses, which are sensory and motor movements. The entire movements of the central nervous system are governed by bodily Air.

The third element is Fire. The source of Fire and light in the solar system is the sun. In the human body, the source of Fire is the metabolism. Fire works in the digestive system. In the gray matter of the brain cells, Fire manifests as intelligence. Fire also activates the retina which perceives light. Thus, body temperature, digestion, the thinking processes and vision are all functions of bodily Fire. All metabolism and enzyme systems are controlled by this element.

Water is the fourth important element in the body. It manifests in the secretions of the digestive juices and the salivary glands, in the mucus membranes and in plasma and cytoplasm. Water is absolutely vital for the functioning of the tissues, organs and various bodily systems. For example, dehydration resulting from diarrhea and vomiting must be treated immediately to protect the patient's life. Because this element is so vital, bodily Water is called the Water of Life.

Earth is the fifth and last element of the cosmos that is present in the microcosm. Life is possible on this plane because Earth holds all living and nonliving substances to its solid surface. In the body, the solid structures — bones, cartilage, nails, muscles, tendons, skin and hair — are derived from Earth.

THE SENSES

The five elements manifest in the functioning of the five senses of man, as well as in certain functions of his physiology. Thus, the five elements are directly related to man's ability to perceive the external environment in which he lives. They are also related, through the senses, to five actions expressing the functions of the sensory organs.

The basic elements — Ether, Air, Fire, Water and Earth — are related to hearing, touch, vision, taste and smell, respectively.

Ether is the medium through which sound is transmitted. Thus, the ethereal element is related to the hearing function. The ear, the organ of hearing, expresses action through the organ of speech, which creates meaningful human sound.

Air is related to the sense of touch; the sensory organ of touch is the skin. The organ of action for the sense of touch is the hand. The skin of the hand is especially sensitive, and the hand is responsible for the actions of holding, giving and receiving.

Fire, which manifests as light, heat and color, is related to vision. The eye, the organ of sight, governs the action of walking and is thus related to the feet. A blind man can walk, but that walking has no definite direction. Eyes give direction to the action of walking.

Water is related to the organ of taste; without water the tongue cannot taste. The tongue is closely related in function to the action of the genitals (penis and clitoris). In Ayurveda, the penis or clitoris

Table 1

The Five Elements, the Organs of the Senses, and Their Actions

ELEMENT	SENSES	SENSE ORGAN	ACTION	ORGAN OF ACTION
Ether	Hearing	Ear	Speech	Organs of Speech (*tongue, vocal cords, mouth*)
Air	Touch	Skin	Holding	Hand
Fire	Seeing	Eyes	Walking	Feet
Water	Taste	Tongue	Procreation	Genitals
Earth	Smell	Nose	Excretion	Anus

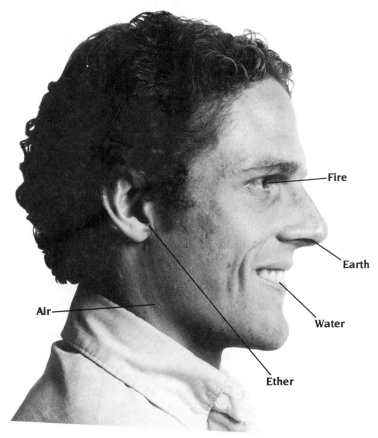

is considered the lower tongue, while the tongue in the mouth is the upper tongue. The person who controls the upper tongue naturally controls the lower tongue.

The Earth element is related to the sense of smell. The nose, the sensory organ of smell, is related in function to the action of the anus, excretion. This relationship is demonstrated by the person who has constipation or an unclean colon: he experiences bad breath and his sense of smell becomes dull.

Ayurveda regards the human body and its sensory experiences as manifestations of cosmic energy expressed in the five basic elements. The ancient *rishis* perceived that these elements sprang from pure Cosmic Consciousness. Ayurveda aims to enable each individual to bring his body into a perfect harmonious relationship with that Consciousness.

CHAPTER III

The Human Constitution

E ther, Air, Fire, Water and Earth, the five basic elements, manifest in the human body as three basic principles, or humors, known as the *tridosha*. From the Ether and Air elements, the bodily air principal called *vata* is manifested. (In Sanskrit terminology, this principle is called *vata dosha*.) The Fire and Water elements manifest together in the body as the fire principle called *pitta*. The Earth and Water elements manifest as the bodily water humor known as *kapha*.

These three elements — *vata - pitta - kapha* — govern all the biological, psychological and physiopathological functions of the body, mind and consciousness. They act as basic constituents and protective barriers for the body in its normal physiological condition; when out of balance, they contribute to disease processes.

The *tridosha* are responsible for the arising of natural urges and for individual preferences in foods: their flavors, temperatures and so on. (See Chapter VIII for a description of the mechanics of these preferences.) They govern the creation, maintenance and destruction of bodily tissue, and the elimination of waste products from the body. They are also responsible for psychological phenomena, including such emotions as fear, anger and greed; and for the highest order of human emotions such as understanding, compassion and love. Thus, the *tridosha* are the foundation of the psychosomatic existence of man.

The basic constitution of each individual is determined at conception. At the time of fertilization, the single male unit, the spermatozoon, unites with the single female element, the ovum. At the moment of this union, the constitution of the individual is determined by the permutations and combinations of bodily air, fire and water that manifest in the parents' bodies.

In general, there are seven types of constitutions: (1) *vata*, (2) *pitta*, (3) *kapha*, (4) *vata-pitta*, (5) *pitta-kapha*, (6) *vata-kapha* and (7) *vata-*

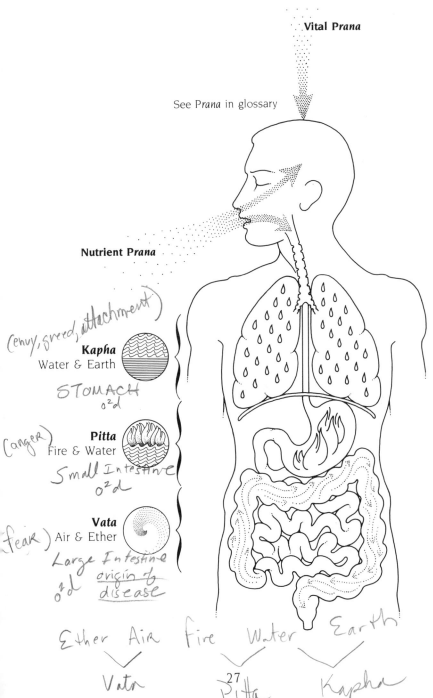

Diagram 1

The Seats of Vata, Pitta, Kapha

Vital Prana

See *Prana* in glossary

Nutrient Prana

(envy, greed, attachment)

Kapha
Water & Earth

STOMACH
o²d

(anger)

Pitta
Fire & Water

Small Intestine
o²d

(fear)

Vata
Air & Ether

Large Intestine
o²d origin of
disease

Ether Air   Fire   Water   Earth

Vata   Pitta   Kapha

27

Chart 2
Functions of Tri-*dosha*

VATA (Air + Space)	PITTA (Fire & Water)	KAPHA (Water + Earth)
Movement	Body Heat	Stability
Breathing	Temperature	Energy
Natural Urges	Digestion	Lubrication
Transformation of Tissues	Perception	Unctuousness
Motor Functions	Understanding	Forgiveness
Sensory Functions	Hunger	Greed
Ungroundedness	Thirst	Attachment
Secretions	Intelligence	Accumulation
Excretions	Anger	Holding
Fear	Hate	Possessiveness
Emptiness	Jealousy	
Anxiety		

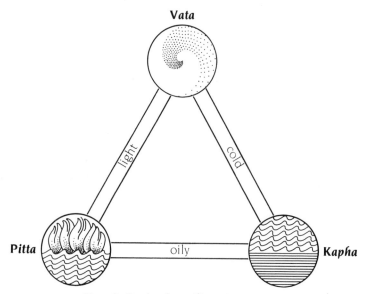

Pitta & Kapha *have oiliness in common*
Pitta & Vata *have lightness in common*
Vata & Kapha *have cold in common*

pitta-kapha. Among these seven general types, there are in-numerable subtle variations that depend upon the percentage of *vata-pitta-kapha* elements in the constitution.

The constitution is called *prakruti* in Sanskrit, a term meaning ''nature,'' ''creativity'' or ''the first creation.'' In the body, the first expression of the basic five elements is the constitution. *The basic constitution of the individual remains unaltered during the lifetime, as it is gene-tically determined. The combination of elements present at birth remains constant. However, the combination of elements that governs the continuous physiopatho-logical changes in the body alters in response to changes in the environment.*

Throughout life, there is a ceaseless interaction between the internal and external environment. The external environment comprises the cosmic forces (macrocosm), while the internal forces (microcosm) are governed by the principles of *vata-pitta-kapha.* A basic principle of healing in Ayurveda holds that one may create balance in the internal forces working in the individual by altering diet and habits of living to counteract changes in his external environment.

UNDERSTANDING TRIDOSHA

According to Ayurveda, the first requirement for healing oneself and others is a clear understanding of the three *dosha,* The concept of *vata-pitta-kapha* is unique to Ayurveda and it holds the potential for revolutionizing the healing systems of the West. How-ever, the concept of the three principles and the Sanskrit words, *vata-pitta-kapha,* are very difficult to translate into Western terms.

Vata is a principle of movement. That which moves is called *vata.* Therefore, *vata* may be translated as the bodily air principle. However, the element of Air in the external atmosphere is not the same as the air in the body. Bodily air, or *vata,* may be characterized as the subtle energy that governs biological movement. This biologi-cal principle of movement engenders all subtle changes in the meta-bolism. *Vata* is formed from the two elements Ether and Air.

Vata governs breathing, blinking of the eyelids, movements in the muscles and tissues, pulsations in the heart; all expansion and contraction, the movements of cytoplasm and the cell membranes, and the movement of the single impulses in nerve cells. Vata also governs such feelings and emotions as freshness, nervousness, fear, anxiety, pain, tremors and spasms. The large intestine, pelvic cavity, bones, skin, ears and thighs are the seats of vata. If the body develops an excess of vata, it will accumulate in these areas.

Pitta is translated as fire, although the term does not literally mean "fire." The fire of a candle or the fire in a fireplace may be seen; however, the bodily heat-energy, the pitta-dosha, which manifests as metabolism is not visible in this way. Pitta governs digestion, absorption, assimilation, nutrition, metabolism, body temperature, skin coloration, the luster of the eyes; and also intelligence and understanding. Psychologically, pitta arouses anger, hate and jealousy. The small intestine, stomach, sweat glands, blood, fat, eyes and skin are the seats of pitta. Pitta is formed from the two elements Fire and Water.

The translation of kapha is biological water, and this bodily principle is formed from the two elements, Earth and Water. Kapha cements the elements in the body, providing the material for physical structure. This dosha maintains body resistance. Water is the main constituent of kapha, and this bodily water is responsible physiologically for biological strength and natural tissue resistance in the body. Kapha lubricates the joints; provides moisture to the skin; helps to heal wounds; fills the spaces in the body; gives biological strength, vigor and stability; supports memory retention; gives energy to the heart and lungs and maintains immunity. Kapha is present in the chest, throat, head, sinuses, nose, mouth, stomach, joints, cytoplasm, plasma and liquid secretions of the body such as mucus. Psychologically, kapha is responsible for emotions of attachment, greed and long-standing envy; it is also expressed in tendencies toward calmness, forgiveness and love. The chest is the seat of kapha.

A balance among the tridosha is necessary for health. For example, the air principle kindles the bodily fire, but water is necessary to control fire, otherwise the bodily fire would burn the tissues. Vata moves kapha and pitta, since kapha and pitta are immobile.

Together, the *tridosha* governs all metabolic activities: anabolism (*kapha*), catabolism (*vata*), and metabolism (*pitta*). When *vata* is out of balance, the metabolism will be disturbed, resulting in excess catabolism, which is the breakdown or deterioration process in the body. When anabolism is greater than catabolism, there is an increased rate of growth and repair of the organs and tissues. Excess *pitta* disturbs metabolism, excess *kapha* increases the rate of anabolism and excess *vata* creates emaciation (catabolism).

In childhood, anabolism and the *kapha* elements are predominant, since this is the time of greatest physical growth. In adulthood, metabolism and the element of *pitta* are most apparent, because at this stage the body is matured and stable. In old age, catabolism and *vata* are most in evidence, as the body begins to deteriorate.

DETERMINING THE INDIVIDUAL CONSTITUTION

The accompanying chart is provided to help the reader determine his or her individual constitution. In addition, a detailed description of the three types of constitutions follows. *It is important to remember that these descriptions reflect the pure aspect of each constitutional element; however, no individual constitution is made up solely of any one element. Rather, each person is a combination of all three elements, with a predominant tendency toward one or more.**

The reader is therefore cautioned not to draw strong or definite conclusions about himself or herself based on these fundamental descriptions. The determination of one's particular constitutional type, using this chart, should serve only to draw general awareness to various areas of life, such as diet, in order to encourage a regimen that will promote good health.

VATA CONSTITUTION

People of *vata* constitution are generally physically underdeveloped. Their chests are flat and their veins and muscle tendons

---

* These characteristic types must be further adjusted according to racial tendencies and cultural preferences, since different races and cultures have natural proclivities for specific body and lifestyle characteristics, *e.g.*, Africans have dark skin and Indians eat hot food.

are visible. The complexion is brown, the skin is cold, rough, dry and cracked. There usually are a few moles present, which tend to be dark.

Vata people generally are either too tall or too short, with thin frames which reveal prominent joints and bone-ends because of poor muscle development. The hair is curly and scanty, the eyelashes are thin and the eyes lusterless. The eyes may be sunken, small, dry, active and the conjunctiva is dry and muddy. The nails are rough and brittle. The shape of the nose is bent and turned-up.

Physiologically, the appetite and digestion are variable. Vata people crave sweet, sour and salty tastes and like hot drinks. The production of urine is scanty and the feces are dry, hard and small in quantity. They have a tendency to perspire less than other constitutional types. Their sleep may be disturbed and they will sleep less than the other types. Their hands and feet are often cold.

These people are creative, active, alert and restless. They talk fast and walk fast but they are easily fatigued.

Psychologically, they are characterized by short memory but quick mental understanding. They will understand something immediately, but will soon forget it. They have little willpower, tend toward mental instability and possess little tolerance, confidence or boldness. Their reasoning power is weak and these people are nervous, fearful and afflicted by much anxiety.

Each constitutional type also exhibits certain patterns in interactions with the external environment. Vata people tend to earn money quickly and also to spend it quickly. Thus, they tend to remain poor.

PITTA CONSTITUTION

These people are of medium height, are slender and body frame may be delicate. Their chests are not as flat as those of vata people and they show a medium prominence of veins and muscle tendons. They have many moles or freckles which are bluish or brownish-red. The bones are not as prominent as in the vata individual. Muscle development is moderate.

The pitta complexion may be coppery, yellowish, reddish or

fair. The skin is soft, warm and less wrinkled than *vata* skin. The hair is thin, silky, red or brownish and there is a tendency toward premature graying of hair and hair loss. The eyes may be gray, green or cooper-brown and sharp; the eyeballs will be of medium prominence. The conjunctiva is moist and copper-colored. The nails are soft. The shape of the nose is sharp and the tip tends to be reddish.

Physiologically, these people have a strong metabolism, good digestion and resulting strong appetites. The person of *pitta* constitution usually takes large quantities of food and liquid. *Pitta* types have a natural craving for sweet, bitter and astringent tastes and enjoy cold drinks. Their sleep is of medium duration but uninterrupted. They produce a large volume of urine and the feces are yellowish, liquid, soft and plentiful. There is a tendency toward excessive perspiring. The body temperature may run slightly high and hands and feet will tend to be warm. *Pitta* people do not tolerate sunlight, heat or hard work well.

Psychologically, *pitta* people have a good power of comprehension; they are very intelligent and sharp and tend to be good orators. They have emotional tendencies toward hate, anger and jealousy.

They are ambitious people who generally like to be leaders. *Pitta* people appreciate material prosperity and they tend to be moderately well-off financially. They enjoy exhibiting their wealth and luxurious possessions.

KAPHA CONSTITUTION

People of *kapha* constitution have well-developed bodies. There is, however, a strong tendency for these individuals to carry excess weight. Their chests are expanded and broad. The veins and tendons of *kapha* people are not obvious because of their thick skin and their muscle development is good. The bones are not prominent.

Their complexions are fair and bright. The skin is soft, lustrous and oily; it is also cold and pale. The hair is thick, dark, soft and wavy. The eyes are dense and black or blue; the white of the eye is generally very white, large and attractive. The conjunctiva does not tend to redness.

Physiologically, *kapha* people have regular appetites, the digestion functions relatively slowly and there is less intake of food. They tend to move slowly. They crave pungent, bitter and astringent foods. Stools are soft and may be pale in color; evacuation is slow. Their perspiration is moderate. Sleep is sound and prolonged. There is a strong vital capacity evidenced by good stamina, and *kapha* people are generally healthy, happy and peaceful.

Psychologically, they tend to be tolerant, calm, forgiving and loving; however, they also exhibit traits of greed, attachment, envy and possessiveness. Their comprehension is slow but definite: once they understand something, that knowledge is retained.

Kapha people tend to be wealthy. They earn money and are good at holding on to it.

Table 2

The Human Constitution (*Prakruti*)

ASPECT OF CONSTITUTION	VATA	PITTA	KAPHA
Frame	Thin	Moderate	Thick
Body Weight	Low	Moderate	Overweight
Skin	Dry, Rough Cool, Brown, Black	Soft, Oily Warm, Fair, Red, Yellowish	Thick, Oily Cool, Pale, White
Hair	Black, Dry, Kinky	Soft, Oily, Yellow, Early Gray, Red	Thick, Oily, Wavy, Dark or Light
Teeth	Protruded, Big and Crooked, Gums Emaciated	Moderate in Size, Soft Gums, Yellowish	Strong, White
Eyes	Small, Dull, Dry, Brown, Black	Sharp, Penetrating, Green, Gray, Yellow	Big, Attractive, Blue, Thick Eyelashes

Table 2, continued

ASPECT OF CONSTITUTION	VATA	PITTA	KAPHA
Appetite	Variable, Scanty	Good, Excessive, Unbearable	Slow but Steady
Taste	Sweet, Sour, Saline	Sweet, Bitter, Astringent	Pungent, Bitter, Astringent
Thirst	Variable	Excessive	Scanty
Elimination	Dry, Hard, Constipated	Soft, Oily, Loose	Thick, Oily, Heavy, Slow
Physical Activity	Very Active	Moderate	Lethargic
Mind	Restless, Active	Aggressive, Intelligent	Calm, Slow
Emotional Temperament	Fearful, Insecure, Unpredictable	Aggressive, Irritable, Jealous	Calm, Greedy, Attached
Faith	Changeable	Fanatic	Steady
Memory	Recent Memory Good, Remote Memory Poor	Sharp	Slow but Prolonged
Dreams	Fearful, Flying Jumping, Running	Fiery, Anger, Violence, War	Watery, River, Ocean, Lake, Swimming, Romantic
Sleep	Scanty, Interrupted	Little but Sound	Heavy, Prolonged
Speech	Fast	Sharp and Cutting	Slow, Monotonous
Financial Status	Poor. Spends Money Quickly on Trifles	Moderate. Spends on Luxuries	Rich. Moneysaver, Spends on Food
Pulse	Thready, Feeble, Moves Like a Snake	Moderate, Jumping Like a Frog	Broad, Slow, Moves Like a Swan

Note: *Circles have been provided next to the aspects for those who wish to determine a general idea of individual constitutional make-up. Mark V for Vata, P for Pitta, or K for Kapha in each circle according to the description best fitting each aspect.*

To experience characteristics different from one's respective doshe *might indicate a derangement of that* doshe.

MENTAL CONSTITUTIONS

On the mental and astral planes, three attributes, or *gunas*, correspond to the three humors that make up the physical constitution. In the Ayurvedic system of medicine, these three attributes provide the basis for distinctions in human temperament and individual differences in psychological and moral dispositions. The three basic attributes are *satva*, *rajas* and *tamas*.

Satva expresses essence, understanding, purity, clarity, compassion and love. *Rajas* implies movement, aggressiveness and extroversion. The *rajas* mind operates on a sensual level. *Tamas* manifests in ignorance, inertia, heaviness and dullness.

People of *satvic* temperament have healthy bodies and their behavior and consciousness are very pure. They believe in the existence of God and are religious and often very holy people.

Individuals of *rajas* temperament are interested in business, prosperity, power, prestige and position. They enjoy wealth and are generally extroverted. They may believe in God but they also may have sudden changes of belief. They are very political.

Tamasic people are lazy, selfish and capable of destroying others. They generally have little respect for others and are not religious. All their activities are egotistical.

The person of *satvic* temperament attains self-realization without much effort while *rajas* and *tamasic* types must make more effort to attain this state.

These three subtle mental energies are responsible for behavioral patterns, which may be altered and improved through the practice of spiritual disciplines such as yoga. The Ayurvedic physician (*vaidya*) can assist in this behavior modification. He is familiar with the functioning of these attributes — *satva*, *rajas* and *tamas* — and he can determine which predominate in the individual by observing behavior and diet. Using these practical clues, he can assist and guide the patient toward a more balanced mental and physical way of living.

Chapter IV
Disease Process

Health is order; disease is disorder. Within the body, there is a constant interaction between order and disorder. The wise man learns to be fully aware of the presence of disorder in his body and then sets about to reestablish order. He understands that order is inherent in disorder and that a return to health is thus possible.

The internal environment of the body is constantly reacting to the external environment. Disorder occurs when these two are out of balance. To change the internal environment in order to bring it into balance with the external environment, one must understand how the disease process occurs within the psychosomatic being. Ayurveda provides explanations of disease that make it possible to restore order and health from disorder and disease.

In Ayurveda, the concept of health is fundamental to the understanding of disease. Dis means "deprived of," and ease means "comfort." Therefore, before discussing disease, we must understand the meaning of comfort or health. A state of health exists when: the digestive fire (*agni*) is in a balanced condition; the bodily humors (*vata-pitta-kapha*) are in equilibrium; the three waste products (urine, feces and sweat) are produced at normal levels and are in balance; the senses are functioning normally; and the body, mind and consciousness are harmoniously working as one. When the balance of any of these systems is disturbed, the disease process begins. Because a balance of the above-mentioned elements and functions is responsible for natural resistance and immunity, even contagious diseases cannot affect the person who is in good health. Thus, imbalances of the body and mind are responsible for physical and psychological pain and misery.

DISEASE CLASSIFICATION
According to Ayurveda, disease may be classified according to

its origin: psychological, spiritual or physical. Disease is also classified according to the site of manifestation: heart, lungs, liver and so forth. The disease process may begin in the stomach or in the intestines, but manifest in the heart or lungs. Thus, disease symptoms may appear in a site other than the locus of origin. Diseases are also classified according to the causative factors and bodily *dosha*: *vata-pitta-kapha*.

DISEASE PRONENESS

The individual constitution determines disease-proneness. For example, people of *kapha* constitution have a definite tendency toward *kapha* diseases. They may experience repeated attacks of tonsillitis, sinusitis, bronchitis and congestion in the lungs. Similarly, individuals of *pitta* constitution are susceptible to gallbladder, bile and liver disorders, hyperacidity, peptic ulcer, gastritis and inflammatory diseases. *Pitta* types also suffer from skin disorders such as hives and rash. *Vata* people are very susceptible to gas, lower back pain, arthritis, sciatica, paralysis and neuralgia. *Vata* diseases have their origin in the large intestine; *pitta* diseases in the small intestine; and *kapha* disorders in the stomach. Imbalanced humors in these areas will create certain signs and symptoms.

The imbalance causing the disease may originate in the consciousness in the form of some negative awareness and it may then manifest in the mind, where the seed of the disease may lie in the deeper subconscious in the form of anger, fear or attachment. These emotions will manifest through the mind into the body. Repressed fear will create derangement of *vata*; anger, excess *pitta*; and envy, greed and attachment, aggravated *kapha*. These imbalances of the *tridosha* affect natural body resistance (the immune system - *agni*) and thus the body becomes susceptible to disease.

Sometimes, the imbalance causing the disease-process may first occur in the body and then manifest in the mind and consciousness. Foods, living habits and environments with attributes similar to those of the *dosha* (humor) will be antagonistic to the bodily tissues. They will create an imbalance that is first manifested on the physical level, and later affects the mind through a disturbance in the *tridosha*.

For instance, disturbed *vata* creates fear, depression and nervousness; excess *pitta* in the body will cause anger, hate and jealousy; aggravated *kapha* creates possessiveness, greed and attachment. Thus, there is a direct connection between diet, habits, environment and emotional disorders.

Impairment of the bodily humors, *vata-pitta-kapha*, creates toxins (*ama*) that are circulated throughout the body. During this circulation, toxins accumulate in the weak areas of the body. If the joint is a weak area, for example, disease will manifest there. What creates these toxins and bodily weaknesses?

KEY TO HEALTH OR DISEASE - 'AGNI'

Agni is the biological fire that governs metabolism. It is similar in its function to *pitta* and can be considered an integral part of the *pitta* system in the body, functioning as a catalytic agent in digestion and metabolism. *Pitta* contains heat-energy which helps digestion. This heat-energy is *agni*. *Pitta* and *agni* are essentially the same with this subtle difference: *pitta* is the container and *agni* is the content.

Pitta manifests in the stomach as the gastric fire, *agni*. *Agni* is acidic in nature and its action breaks down food and stimulates digestion. *Agni* is also subtly related to the movement of *vata* because bodily air enkindles bodily fire. In every tissue and cell, *agni* is present and necessary for maintaining the nutrition of the tissues and the maintenance of the auto-immune mechanism. *Agni* destroys micro-organisms, foreign bacteria and toxins in the stomach and small and large intestines. In this way, it protects the flora in these organs.

Longevity depends upon *agni*. Intelligence, understanding, perception and comprehension are also the functions of *agni*. The color of the skin is maintained by *agni*, and the enzyme system and metabolism totally depend upon *agni*. As long as *agni* is functioning properly, the processes of breaking down food and absorbing and assimilating it into the body will operate smoothly.

When *agni* becomes impaired because of an imbalance in the *tridosha*, the metabolism is drastically affected. The body's resistance and immune system are impaired. Food components remain undigested and unabsorbed. They accumulate in the large intestine turning into a heterogeneous, foul-smelling, sticky substance. This material, which is called *ama*, clogs the intestines and other channels, such as capillaries and blood vessels. It eventually undergoes many chemical changes which create toxins. These toxins are absorbed into the blood and enter the general circulation. They eventually accumulate in the weaker parts of the body, where they create contraction, clogging, stagnation and weakness of the organs and reduce the immune mechanism of the respective tissues. Finally, a disease condition manifests in the affected organs and is identified as arthritis, diabetes, heart disease and so on. toxins

 The root of all disease is *ama*. There are many causes for the development of *ama*. For example, whenever incompatible foods are ingested, *agni* will be directly affected as a result of the toxins, or *ama*, created from these poorly digested foods. If the tongue is coated with a white film, this symptom indicates that *ama* exists in the large intestine, small intestine or stomach, depending upon which part of the tongue is coated. (See section and diagram on tongue diagnosis in Chapter VI.)

Ama develops when *agni*'s function is retarded; however, overactive *agni* is also detrimental. When *agni* becomes hyperactive, the digestive process burns away, through overcombustion, the normal biological nutrients in the food and emaciation results. This condition also lowers the body's immunity.

REPRESSED EMOTIONS
Toxins are also created by emotional factors. Repressed anger, for example, completely changes the flora of the gallbladder, bile duct and small intestine and aggravates *pitta*, causing inflamed patches on the mucous membranes of the stomach and small intestine. In a similar manner, fear and anxiety alter the flora of the large intestine. As a result, the belly becomes bloated with gas, which accumulates in pockets of the large intestine causing pain. Often this pain is mistaken for heart or liver problems. Because of the ill-effects of repression, it is recommended that neither the emotions

nor any bodily urge, such as coughing, sneezing and passing gas, should be repressed.

Repressed emotions create an imbalance of *vata* which in turn affects *agni*, the body's auto-immune response. When *agni* is low, an abnormal immune reaction may occur. This reaction may cause allergies to certain substances, such as pollen, dust and flower scents.*

Because allergies are closely related to the immune responses of the body, individuals who are born with an abnormal immune reaction often suffer from allergies. For example, a person born with a *pitta* constitution will be naturally sensitive to hot, spicy foods which aggravate *pitta*. In the same way, repressed *pitta* emotions such as hate and anger also may increase the hypersensitivity to those foods that aggravate *pitta*.

People with *kapha* constitutions are very sensitive to foods that aggravate *kapha*. In such individuals, *kaphagenic* foods such as dairy products produce disturbances like cough, cold, congestion and wheezing. Individuals who repress *kapha* emotions such as attachment and greed will have allergic reactions to *kapha* foods.

Ayurveda recommends that emotions be observed with detachment and then allowed to dissipate. When emotions are repressed, that repression will cause disturbances in the mind and eventually in the functioning of the body.

THE THREE MALAS

Imbalances in other bodily systems, such as the waste systems, also may result in disease. The body produces three waste products, or *malas*: feces, which are solid; and urine and sweat, which are liquid. The production and elimination of these is absolutely vital to health. Urine and feces are formed during the digestive process in the large intestine, where assimilation, absorption and discrimination between essential and nonessential substances take

---

* Because of their origin in repressed emotion, allergies cannot be radically cured by the use of antihistamines.

Intestinal parasites are another cause of allergy. For instance, if threadworms, roundworms or amoebas are present in the large intestine, an allergy to pollen grains might result.

place. Feces are carried to the rectum for evacuation; urine is carried to the kidneys for filtration and then stored in the bladder for elimination; and sweat is eliminated through the pores of the skin.

Though they are considered bodily waste products, the urine and feces are not strictly waste. They are, in fact, to some extent essential to the physiological functioning of their respective organs. For example, feces supply nutrition through intestinal tissues: many nutrients remain in the feces after digestion. Later, after these are absorbed, the feces are eliminated.

Feces also give strength to the large intestine and maintain its tone. If a person has no feces, the intestine will collapse. A person who suffers from constipation lives longer than one who suffers from diarrhea. If diarrhea continues for fifteen days, death will follow. However, one can experience prolonged constipation and live, though it will cause problems in the bodily systems. Constipation creates distention and discomfort, flatulence and pains in the body, headache and bad breath.

The urinary system removes the water, salt and nitrogenous wastes of the body. Urine is formed in the large intestine. This waste product helps to maintain the normal concentration of water electrolytes within the body fluids. The functioning of this *mala* depends upon the water intake, diet, environmental temperature, mental state and physical condition of the individual.

The color of the urine depends upon the diet. If the patient has a fever, which is a *pitta* disorder, the urine will become darkish yellow or brownish. Jaundice, which is also a *pitta* disorder, causes dark yellow urine. Bile pigmentation may give the urine a greenish color. Excess *pitta* may create high acidity in the urine. The substances that stimulate urination, such as tea, coffee and alcohol, also aggravate *pitta*.

If the body retains water, the urine will be scanty and this water will accumulate in the tissues. This condition, in turn, will affect the blood and increase the blood pressure. So, balanced urine production is important for the maintenance of blood pressure and volume.

Ayurvedic texts state that human urine is a natural laxative that

Chart 3
Examination of Urine

The body fluids, such as blood (*rakta*) and lymph (*rasa*) serve to carry wastes (*malas*) away from the tissues that produce them. The urinary system removes water (*kleda*), salt and nitrogenous wastes (*dhatu malas*). The urinary system also helps to maintain the normal concentration of water electrolytes within the body fluids. It helps to regulate the volume of body fluid and aids in the control of red blood cell production and blood pressure. Thus. the urine helps to maintain the balance of the three humours — *vata-pitta-kapha* — and water.

Clinical Examination of Urine: In a clean vessel, collect the early morning urine in mid-stream. Observe the color. If the color is blackish-brown, this indicates a Vata disorder; if the color is dark-yellow, a Pitta disorder. Also, when there is constipation or the body has less intake of water, urine will be dark yellow. If the urine is cloudy, there is a Kapha disorder. A red color in the urine indicates a blood disorder.

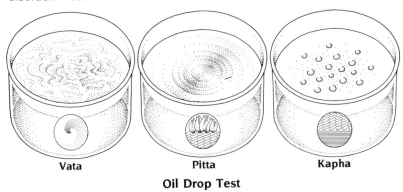

| Vata | Pitta | Kapha |

Oil Drop Test

With a dropper, place one drop of sesame oil in a sample of urine. If the drop spreads immediately, the physical disorder is easy to cure. If the drop sinks to the middle of the urine sample, this indicates illness is difficult to cure. If the drop sinks to the bottom, illness may be very difficult to cure.

If drop spreads on the surface in wave-like movements, this indicates Vata disorder. If drop spreads on the surface with multiple colors visible like a rainbow, this indicates Pitta disorder. If drop breaks up into pearl-like droplets on the surface of urine, this indicates Kapha disorder.

Normal urine has a typical uremic smell. However, if the urine has a foul odor, this indicates that there are toxins in the system. An acidic smell which creates a burning sensation indicates excess Pitta. A sweet smell of urine indicates a possible diabetic condition. In this condition, the individual experiences goose bumps on the skin while passing urine. Gravel in the urine indicates the likelihood of stones in the urinary tract.

detoxifies poisons in the system and helps absorption in the large intestine as well as the elimination of feces. If one takes a cup of urine (passed in midstream) every morning it will help to cleanse and detoxify the large intestine.

Perspiration is a by-product of fatty tissue. Sweating is necessary to regulate the body temperature. Sweat keeps the skin soft, maintains the flora of the pores of the skin and also maintains skin elasticity and tone.

Excessive sweating is a disorder that can create fungal infection and reduces the natural resistance of the skin. Insufficient sweating will also reduce the resistance of the skin and it will cause the skin to become rough and scaly, creating dandruff.

There is a special relationship between the skin and the kidneys since the excretion of watery wastes is primarily the function of these two organs. Thus, perspiration is indirectly related to the formation of urine. Like urine, perspiration is related to *pitta*. In summer people perspire profusely, but their urination is reduced because waste products are eliminated through perspiration. In winter, many people perspire less and urinate more.

Excessive urination may cause too little perspiration production and excessive perspiring may result in a scanty volume of urine. Thus, it is necessary that the production of perspiration and urine be in balance. Diabetes, psoriasis, dermatitis and ascites (dropsy) are examples of diseases resulting from an imbalance of perspiration and urine in the body.

Excessive perspiration reduces body temperature and creates dehydration. In the same way, too much urination also creates dehydration and also will cause coldness of the hands and feet.

THE SEVEN DHATUS

The human body consists of seven basic and vital tissues called *dhatus*. The Sanskrit word *dhatu* means "constructing element." These seven are responsible for the entire structure of the body. The *dhatus* maintain the functions of the different organs, systems and vital parts of the body. They play a very important role in the development and nourishment of the body.

The *dhatus* are also part of the biological protective mechanism. With the help of *agni*, they are responsible for the immune mechanism. When one *dhatu* is defective, it affects the successive *dhatu*, as each *dhatu* receives its nourishment from the previous *dhatu*. The following are the seven most important *dhatus* in serial order:

1) *Rasa* (plasma) contains nutrients from digested food and nourishes all the tissues, organs and systems.
2) *Rakta* (blood) governs oxygenation in all tissues and vital organs and maintains life.
3) *Mamsa* (muscle) covers the delicate vital organs, performs the movements of the joints and maintains the physical strength of the body.
4) *Meda* (fat) maintains the lubrication and oiliness of all the tissues.
5) *Asthi* (bone) gives support to the body structure.
6) *Majja* (marrow and nerves) fills up the bony spaces and carries motor and sensory impulses.
7) *Shukra* and *Artav* (reproductive tissues) contain the ingredients of all tissues and are responsible for reproduction.

The seven *dhatus* are understood in a natural, biological, serial order of manifestation. The post-digestion of food, called 'nutrient plasma,' *ahara rasa*, contains the nutrition for all the *dhatus*. This 'nutrient plasma' is transformed and nourished with the help of heat, called *dhatu agni*, of each respective *dhatu*.

Rasa is transformed into *rakta*, which is further manifested into *mamsa*, *meda*, etc. This transformation results from three basic actions: irrigation (nutrients are carried to the seven *dhatus* through the blood vessels); selectivity (each *dhatu* extracts the nutrients it requires in order to perform its physiological functions); and direct transformation (as the nutritional substances pass through each *dhatu*, the food for the formation of each subsequent *dhatu* is produced). These three processes — irrigation, selectivity and transformation — operate simultaneously in the formation of the seven *dhatus*. The *dhatus* are nourished and transformed in order to maintain the normal physiological functions of the different tissues, organs and systems.

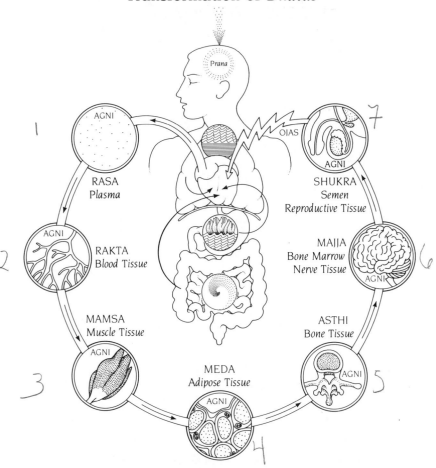

Chart 4
The Circulation of Nutrients and Transformation of D*hatus*

THE SEVEN DHATUS: 1) RASA (*plasma*)—maintains functions of menstruation (ARTAVA) in the uterus and lactation (STANYA) in the mammary glands. **2) RAKTA** (*blood tissue or red blood cells*)—maintains muscle tendons (KANDARA) and blood vessels (SIRA). **3) MAMSA** (*muscle tissue*)-maintains flat muscle (SNAYU) and the skin (TWACHA). **5) MEDA** (*adipose tissue*)—maintains subcutaneous fat (VASA) and function of sweat (SWEDA). **5) ASTHI** (*bone tissue*)—maintains teeth (DANTA), nails (NAKHA) and hair (KESHA). **6) MAJJA** (*bone marrow, nerve tissue*)—maintains function of lacrimal secretion (AKSHIVIT SNEHA). **7) SHUKRA** (*semen, reproductive tissue*)—maintains function of sexual organs.

When there is a disorder in the balance of *vata-pitta-kapha*, the *dhatus* are directly affected. The disturbed *dosha* (*vata*, *pitta* or *kapha*) and defective *dhatus* are always directly involved in the disease process. Health of the *dhatus* can be maintained by taking steps to keep *vata-pitta-kapha* in balance through a proper diet, exercise and rejuvenation program.

CHAPTER V
Attributes

अ, ह Guna

Ayurveda encompasses a subtle medical science of attributes or qualities. These attributes are also called *gunas*. Charak, the great Ayurvedic physician, found that all organic and inorganic substances, as well as all thoughts and actions have definite attributes. These attributes contain potential energy while the actions express kinetic energy. Attributes and actions are closely related since the potential energy of the attributes eventually becomes action or kinetic energy. According to Ayurveda, there are twenty basic attributes. The accompanying table shows these twenty attributes and their actions.

After close observation of the universe and man, Charak categorized the twenty basic attributes into ten antagonistic pairs (*e.g.*, hot and cold; slow and fast; dull and sharp; wet and dry). These opposite forces function together. The universe as a whole is the manifestation of the two most basic opposites, male and female energy. Thus it is possible to understand the universe in terms of the interactions of opposing forces that manifest as the basic attributes.

Vata, pitta and *kapha* each have their own attributes, and substances having similar attributes will tend to aggravate the related bodily humor by the law of like-increases-like. For instance, the summer season has attributes similar to those of *pitta* — hot, dry, light, motile and penetrating. Naturally, in the summer, *pitta* in the body will be aggravated. *Vata* is light, subtle, dry, mobile, rough and cold. So, in the fall season, which also exhibits these attributes, *vata* will tend to be aggravated in the human constitution. Lastly, *kapha* is liquid, heavy, cold, sticky and cloudy; so in winter when these characteristics predominate in the external environment, internal *kapha* tends to be aggravated.

If one continually takes substances with attributes opposite to those in their body, those opposite attributes will become dominant and may result in derangement. For instance, a *vata* individual naturally has an excess of light attributes. However, if the individual continually ingests heavy *kapha*-causing foods, which inhibit the light attributes of the body, over a period of time that individual's bodily attributes will be altered from *vata* (light) to *kapha* (heavy). In this way, the attributes of the body may be changed, in spite of the inherent natural tendencies of the constitution.

To understand and appreciate the Ayurvedic concept of attributes, one should meditate deeply upon them. The examination of attributes is a very subtle experience and it demands constant awareness. If one eats hot, spicy chilis, for instance, what do the senses reflect? Because of the sharp and penetrating action of this food, one immediately experiences such bodily sensations as heat, sweating and a burning sensation in the mouth. Also on the following day, the urine and feces might create a burning sensation.

The concepts governing the pharmacology, therapeutics and food preparation in Ayurveda are based on the action and reaction of the twenty attributes to and upon one another. Through understanding of these attributes, balance of the *tridosha* may be maintained.

+ implementing

Inherent natural tendencies

49

Table 3
The Twenty Attributes (Gunas)
and Their Actions *Pairs of Opposites*

1. **Heavy** (Guru) — Increases Kapha; decreases Vata and Pitta. Increases bulk nutrition, heaviness. Creates dullness, lethargy.

2. **Light** (Laghu) — Increases Vata, Pitta and Agni; decreases Kapha. Helps digestion, reduces bulk, cleanses. Creates freshness, alertness, ungroundedness.

3. **Slow** (Manda) — Increases Kapha; decreases Vata and Pitta. Creates sluggishness, slow action, relaxation, dullness.

4. **Sharp** (Tikshna) — Increases Vata and Pitta; decreases Kapha. Creates ulcers, perforation, has immediate effect on body. Promotes sharpness, quick understanding.

5. **Cold** (Shita) — Increases Vata and Kapha; decreases Pitta. Creates cold, numbness, unconsciousness, contraction, fear, insensitivity.

6. **Hot** (Ushna) — Increases Pitta and Agni; decreases Vata and Kapha. Promotes heat, digestion, cleansing, expansion, inflammation, anger, hate.

7. **Oily** (Snigdha) — Increases Pitta and Kapha; decreases Vata and Agni. Creates smoothness, moisture, lubrication, vigor. Promotes compassion, love.

8. **Dry** (Ruksha) — Increases Vata and Agni; decreases Pitta and Kapha. Increases dryness, absorption, constipation, nervousness.

9. **Slimy** (Slakshna) — Increases Pitta and Kapha; decreases Vata and Agni. Decreases roughness. Increases smoothness, love, care.

10. **Rough** (Khara) — Increases Vata and Agni; decreases Pitta and Kapha. Causes cracking of skin, bones, creates carelessness, rigidity.

11. **Dense** (Sandra) — Increases Kapha; decreases Vata, Pitta and Agni. Promotes solidity, density, strength.

12. **Liquid** (Drava) — Increases Pitta and Kapha; decreases Vata and Agni. Dissolves, liquifies. Promotes salivation, compassion, cohesiveness.

13. **Soft** (Mrudu) — Increases Pitta and Kapha; decreases Vata and Agni. Creates softness, delicacy, relaxation, tenderness, love, care.

14. **Hard** (Kathina) — Increases Vata and Kapha; decreases Pitta and Agni. Increases hardness, strength, rigidity, selfishness, callousness, insensitivity.

15. **Static** (Sthira) — Increases Kapha; decreases Vata, Pitta and Agni. Promotes stability, obstruction, support, constipation, faith.

16. **Mobile** (Chala) — Increases Vata, Pitta and Agni; decreases Kapha. Promotes motion, shakiness, restlessness, lack of faith.

50

17. **Subtle** (*Sukshma*) — Increases Vata, Pitta and Agni; decreases Kapha. Pierces. Penetrates subtle capillaries. Increases emotions, feeling.

18. **Gross** (*Sthula*) — Increases Kapha; decreases Vata, Pitta and Agni. Causes obstruction, obesity.

19. **Cloudy** (*Avila*) — Increases Kapha; decreases Vata, Pitta and Agni. Heals fractures. Causes unclearness, lack of perception.

20. **Clear** (*Vishada*) — Increases Vata, Pitta and Agni; decreases Kapha. Pacifies. Creates isolation, diversion.

Table 4
Attributes of the Tri-*dosha*

VATA	**PITTA**	**KAPHA**
dry	oily	heavy
light	penetrating	slow
cold	hot	cold
rough	light	oily
subtle	mobile	slimy
mobile	liquid	dense
clear	sour smell	soft
dispersing		static

Elements of the Tri-Dosha

VATA	**PITTA**	**KAPHA**
Air + Ether	Fire + Water	Earth + Water

Ether + AiR   *fire*   *water + Earth*

51

CHAPTER VI

Diagnosis

I n the West, the term *diagnosis* generally refers to identification of the disease after it has manifested. However, in Ayurveda, the concept of diagnosis implies a moment-to-moment monitoring of the interactions between order (health) and disorder (disease) in the body. The disease process is a reaction between the bodily humors and the tissues. The symptoms of disease are always related to derangement of the balance of the *tridosha*. Once we understand the nature of the imbalance, balance may be reestablished through treatment.

Ayurveda teaches very precise methods for understanding the disease process before any overt signs of the disease have manifested. By detecting early symptoms of imbalance and disease reaction in the body, one can determine the nature of future bodily reactions. Day-to-day observation of the pulse, tongue, face, eyes, nails and lips provide subtle indicators. Through these, the student of Ayurveda can learn what pathological processes are occurring in the body, which organs are impaired and where *dosha* and toxins have accumulated. Thus, by checking the body's indicators regularly, pathological symptoms can be detected early and preventative measures taken. Ayurveda teaches that the patient is a living book and, for understanding and physical well-being, he or she must be read daily.

EXAMINATION OF THE RADIAL PULSE

As the diagram shows, the radial pulse is felt with the first three fingers: the index, middle and ring fingers. To make a complete examination of the pulse, the doctor faces the patient and takes the pulse of each of his patient's wrists. The indicators of the pulse vary from the left to right side, so it is best to check the pulse on both sides of the body. The pulse should not be taken after exertion, massage, eating, bathing or sex. The pulse will also be affected by

Diagram 2
(Nadi) Pulse Diagnosis

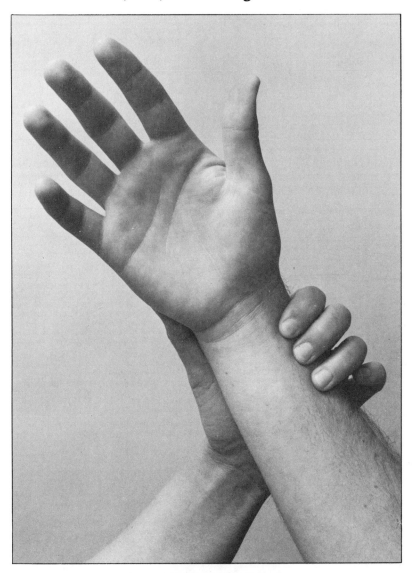

EXAMINATION OF PULSE

Keep the arm slightly bent, and flex the wrist slightly. Place the three fingers superficially to feel the throbbings of the pulse. Slightly loosen the fingers to feel different movements of the pulse.

IDENTIFICATION OF THE PULSE

Vata

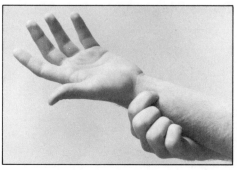

Fast, Narrow, Feeble, Cool, Irregular.

Rate is 80-100 beats per minute.

1) The placement of the index finger denotes the pulse of Vata. When this pulse predominates, the index finger feels the throbbing more strongly. Also, the pulse feels like the movement of a snake, quick and slithery.

Pitta

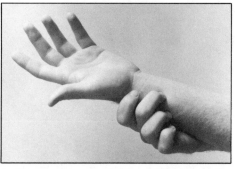

Jumping, Excited, Prominent, Hot, Moderate, Regular.

Rate is 70-80 beats per minute.

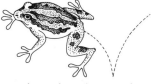

2) The placement of the middle finger denotes the pulse of Pitta. When this pulse predominates, the middle finger is strongest. It is active and jumpy like the movement of a frog.

Kapha

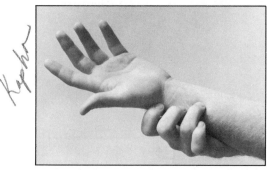

Slow, Strong, Steady, Soft, Broad, Regular, Warm.

Rate is 60-70 beats per minute.

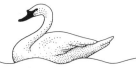

3) The placement of the ring finger denotes the pulse of Kapha. When this pulse predominates, the ring finger feels strongest. This pulse is slow and resembles the floating of a swan.

Diagram 3

Pulse Points

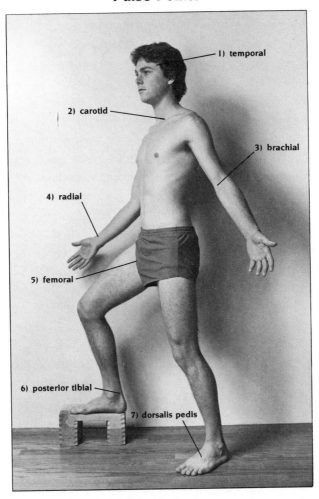

1) temporal

2) carotid

3) brachial

4) radial

5) femoral

6) posterior tibial

7) dorsalis pedis

THE PULSE MAY BE CHECKED: 1) At the temporal artery, just above the temple on the side of the head. 2) At the carotid artery, on the side of the neck above the clavicle. 3) At the brachial artery, on the inside of the arm above the elbow. 4) At the radial artery, on the wrist. 5) At the femoral artery, on the inside front of the leg where it joins the pelvis. 6) At the posterior tibial artery, on the foot behind the ankle. 7) At the dorsalis pedis artery, on the top of the foot.

sitting near heat or by taking strenuous exercise. The pulse may be taken at other points on the body as well. (See pulse points diagram.)

To check your own pulse, keep your arm and wrist slightly flexed. Place your three fingers lightly on the wrist just below the radial bone (wrist bone) and feel the throbbing of the pulse. Then decrease the pressure of your fingers slightly to sense varying movements of the pulse.

The position of the index finger denotes the place of the *vata dosha*. When *vata* is predominant in the constitution, the index finger will feel the pulse strongly. It will be irregular and thin, moving in waves like the motion of a serpent. This type of pulse is therefore called the "snake" pulse and it indicates aggravated *vata* in the body.

The resting place of the middle finger denotes the pulse of the *pitta dosha*. When *pitta* is predominant in the constitution, the pulse will be stronger under the middle finger. It will feel active and excited and will move like the jumping of a frog. Hence, it is called the "frog" pulse. This pulse denotes aggravated *pitta*.

When *kapha* is predominant, the throbbing of the pulse under the ring finger is most noticeable. The pulse feels strong and its movement resembles the floating of a swan. It is called the "swan" pulse.

Not only the constitution, but also the status of the body's organs can be determined by examination of the superficial and deep pulsations. The beats of the pulse not only correspond to the heartbeat, but they also reveal something about the important meridians that are connecting *pranic* currents of energy in the body. These currents circulate through the blood, passing through the vital organs such as the liver, kidney, heart and brain. By feeling the superficial and deep pulsations, the sensitive examiner can detect the conditions of these various organs. Each finger rests on a meridian of the element associated with the *dosha* of that place. (See hand chart.) For example, the index finger which rests on the *vata dosha* detects bodily air; the middle finger which touches on *pitta* detects fire; and the ring finger which feels the *kapha* pulse, water.

The index finger rests on the patient's right wrist at the site for feeling the activity of the large intestine with a superficial touch;

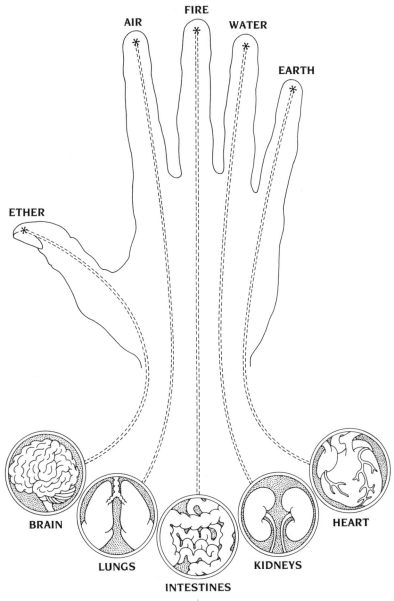

Diagram 4

The Meridians and
The Basic Five Elements

AIR

FIRE

WATER

EARTH

ETHER

BRAIN

LUNGS

INTESTINES

KIDNEYS

HEART

BLIKH

Diagram 5

The Pulse and the Organs

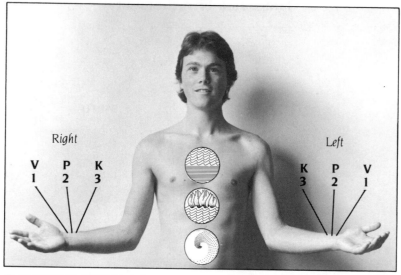

	Right					Left	
V	**P**	**K**			**K**	**P**	**V**
1	**2**	**3**			**3**	**2**	**1**

SUPERFICIAL TOUCH: 1) Large Intestine, 2) Gall Bladder, 3) Pericardium. DEEP TOUCH: 1) Lung, 2) Liver, 3) *Vata-Pitta-Kapha*.

SUPERFICIAL TOUCH: 1) Small Intestine, 2) Stomach, 3) Bladder. DEEP TOUCH: 1) Heart, 2) Spleen, 3) Kidney.

PULSE SHOULD NOT BE CHECKED: 1) After Massage, 2) After Taking Food or Alcohol, 3) After Sunbathing, 4) After Sitting Close to a Fire, 5) After Hard Physical Labor, 6) After Sex, 7) While Hungry, 8) While Taking a Bath.

PULSE RATE IN RELATION TO AGE: 1) Baby in the Womb—160, 2) Baby after Birth—140, 3) Birth to One Year—130, 4) One to Two Years—100, 5) Three to Seven Years—95, 6) Eight to Fourteen Years—80, 7) Adult Average—72, 8) Old Age—65, 9) Sickness—120, 10) Time of Death—160.

when firmer, deeper pressure is applied, the activity of the lungs may be sensed. If very prominent throbbing is felt when the index finger on the right side is applied superficially, then *vata* is aggravated in the large intestine; if the deep pulse is strong and throbbing, there is congestion in the lungs. The middle finger resting on the right wrist can detect the status of the gallbladder with superficial touch and the liver with deeper pressure. The ring finger senses the pericardium (outer covering of the heart) when applied superficially; and, with a deep touch, the harmonious relationship of *vata-pitta-kapha* is detected.

The index finger resting superficially on the patient's left wrist monitors the activity of the small intestine, while the heart is monitored by deep pressure. With superficial pressure of the middle finger, the activity of the stomach is observed; and deep pressure reveals the status of the spleen. The ring finger applied superficially reveals the condition of the bladder while deep pressure checks the functioning of the kidneys. To learn this technique of examination of the pulse requires attention and day-to-day practice.

You can feel the variations in your pulse at different times of the day. You can also note changes in the pulse after urination, when you are hungry or when you feel anger. Observing such changes, you will begin to learn how to read the pulse.

TONGUE DIAGNOSIS

The tongue is the organ of taste and speech. We perceive taste through the tongue when it is wet; a dry tongue cannot perceive taste. The tongue is also the vital organ of speech, used to convey in words, thoughts, concepts, ideas and feelings. Examination of this important organ reveals the totality of what is happening in the body.

Look at your tongue in the mirror. Observe the size, shape, contour, surface, margins and color. If the color is pale, there is an anemic condition or lack of blood in the body. If the color is yellowish, excess bile exists in the gallbladder or there is a liver disorder. If the color is blue (provided one has not eaten blueberries), there is some defect in the heart.

As shown in the diagram, different parts of the tongue are related to different organs in the body. If there are discolorations, depressions or elevations on certain areas of the tongue, the respective organs are defective. For example, if you see the im-

Diagram 6
Tongue Diagnosis (Jihva)

CONDITIONS: A discoloration and/or sensitivity of a particular area of the tongue indicates a disorder in the organ corresponding to that area (see diagram). A whitish tongue indicates *Kapha* derangement and mucus accumulation; a red or yellow-green tongue indicates *Pitta* derangement; and a black-to-brown coloration indicates *Vata* derangement. A dehydrated tongue is symptomatic of a decrease in the *dhatu Rasa* (plasma), while a pale tongue indicates a decrease in the *dhatu Rakta* (red blood cells).

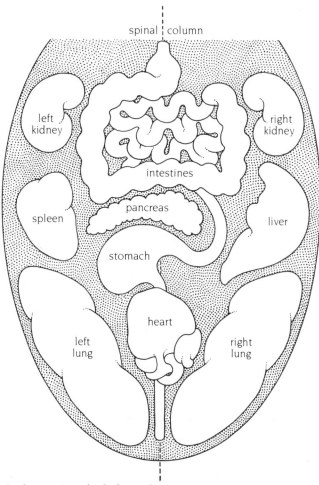

Note: *This diagram is used to look at one's own tongue in a mirror. It is a mirror image.*

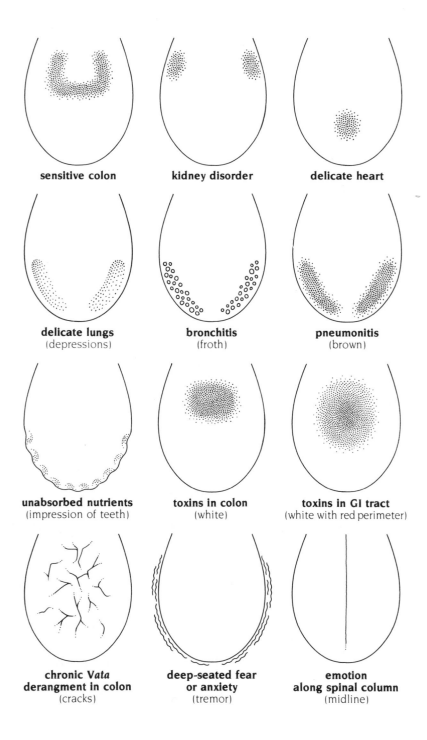

sensitive colon

kidney disorder

delicate heart

delicate lungs
(depressions)

bronchitis
(froth)

pneumonitis
(brown)

unabsorbed nutrients
(impression of teeth)

toxins in colon
(white)

toxins in GI tract
(white with red perimeter)

**chronic Vata
derangment in colon**
(cracks)

**deep-seated fear
or anxiety**
(tremor)

**emotion
along spinal column**
(midline)

Diagram 6, continued

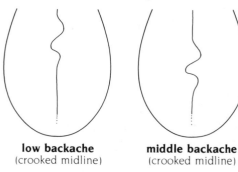

low backache
(crooked midline)

middle backache
(crooked midline)

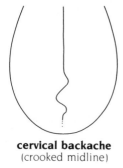

cervical backache
(crooked midline)

pressions of the teeth along the margin of the tongue, this indicates poor intestinal absorption.

A coating covering the tongue indicates toxins in the stomach, small intestine or large intestine. If only the posterior part is coated, toxins are present in the large intestine; if the middle of the tongue is coated, toxins are present in the stomach and small intestine.

A line down the middle of the tongue indicates that emotions are being held along the vertebral column. If this line is curved, it may indicate a deformity in the curvature of the spine.

FACIAL DIAGNOSIS

The face is the mirror of the mind. The lines and wrinkles in your face are revealing. If disorder and disease are present, they will be indicated on the face. Observe the different parts of your face carefully in the mirror. Horizontal wrinkling on the forehead indicates you have deep-seated worries and anxieties. A vertical line between the eyebrows on the right side indicates your emotions are repressed in the liver. A vertical line between the eyebrows on the left side indicates your spleen is holding in emotions.

When the lower eyelids are full and puffy, it indicates that the kidneys are impaired. A butterfly-like discoloration on the nose or on the cheeks just below the kidney region (see accompanying dia-

Diagram 7

Facial Diagnosis

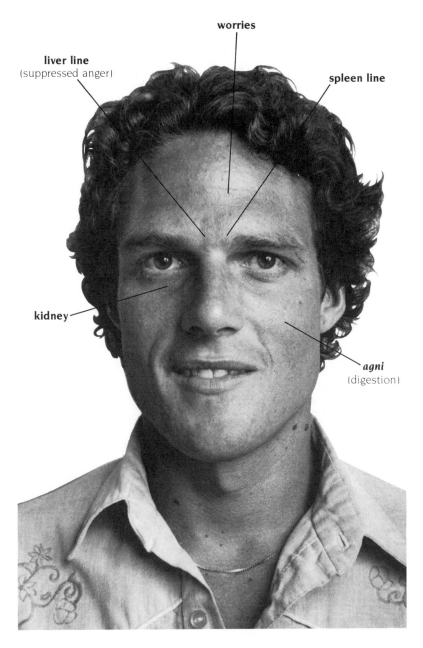

worries

liver line
(suppressed anger)

spleen line

kidney

agni
(digestion)

gram) means the body is not absorbing iron or folic acid and the digestive metabolism is not working properly because of low *agni*.

Generally, a person of *vata* constitution cannot gain weight. Therefore, his cheeks become flat and sunken. A person whose metabolism is slow (*kapha* constitution) will retain water, fat and the cheeks will be plump.

The shape of the nose can indicate the constitution. A sharp nose may denote *pitta*; a blunt nose, *kapha*; and a crooked nose, *vata*.

LIP DIAGNOSIS

As with the other features of the body (*e.g.*, tongue, nails, face, eyes), the lips, too, reflect the health or disease of the various physical organs.

One should observe the size, shape, surface, color and contour of the lips. If they are dry and rough, this indicates dehydration or a *vata* derangement. Nervousness and fear also create dryness and tremors of the lips. In anemia, the lips become pale. As a result of chronic smoking, the lips become blackish-brown. Repeated attacks of inflammatory patches along the margins of the lips indicates the presence of herpes and a chronic *pitta* derangement. If there are multiple pale brown spots on the lips, poor digestion or worms in the colon are indicated. If a jaundice condition exists, the lips become yellow. In heart disorders, because of lack of oxygen, the lips become blue. Discoloration of the various areas of the lips indicates a disorder of the respective organ. (See diagram.)

NAIL DIAGNOSIS

According to Ayurveda, the nails are a waste product of the bones. Look at the size, shape, surface and contour of your nails. Also, observe whether they are flexible, soft and tender, or brittle and easily broken.

If the nails are dry, crooked, rough and break easily, *vata* predominates in the body. If the nails are soft, pink, tender, easily bent and slightly glistening, *pitta* predominates. When the nails are thick, strong, soft and very shiny with a uniform contour, then *kapha* predominates.

Diagram 8

Lip Diagnosis (Ostha)

CONDITIONS: Vata lips are thin and dry, Pitta lips are red, and Kapha lips are thick and oily. Dry or cracked lips indicate dehydration and Vata derangement. Pale lips are symptomatic of anemia. Brown spots are a sign of chronic indigestion and can mean the presence of worms in the colon. Herpes blisters or ulcers on the lips indicate Pitta derangement. Tremors of the lips are a sign of fear or anxiety.

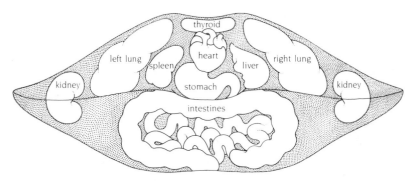

Note: This diagram is used to look at one's own lips in a mirror. It is a mirror image.

Longitudinal lines on the nails indicate malabsorption in the digestive system. Transverse grooves on the nails reveal defective nutrition or a long-standing illness.

Sometimes the nails become prominent, convex and bulbous like a drumstick. This condition, which is called clubbing, indicates delicate lungs and heart. When the nail is spoon-shaped and concave so that it will hold a drop of water an iron deficiency exists. White spots on the nail indicate a zinc or calcium deficiency.

Pale nails indicate anemia. Undue redness shows an excess of red blood cells. Yellow nails indicate a delicate liver or jaundice. Blue nails show a weak heart.

Each finger and the thumb correspond to an organ of the body. The thumbnail corresponds to the brain and skull and the index finger to the lungs. The middle finger relates to the small in-

BL I KH

65 Thumb, index, middle, ring, pinky

Diagram 9
Nail Diagnosis

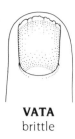

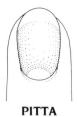

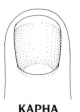

VATA
brittle

PITTA
soft, pink, tender

KAPHA
thick, strong oily

CONDITIONS: Coloration of the nail can denote a particular disorder. If the nail is pale, anemia is indicated. A yellow nail is a sign of a delicate liver, while a blue nail is symptomatic of delicate lungs and heart. If the luna (the crescent at the base of the nail) is blue, a disturbed liver is indicated. A red luna is a sign of cardiac failure.

nervousness
Vata derangement
(bitten nail)

malnutrition
Agni derangement
(stepped surface)

malabsorption
Vata derangement
(longitudinal striations)

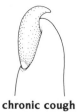

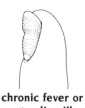

delicate heart & lungs
poor *Prana*
(clubbed nail)

chronic cough
Kapha derangement
(parrot beak)

**chronic fever or
long-standing illness**
(transverse groove)

chronic lung infection
Kapha derangement
(bump at end of nail)

**calcium or zinc
deficiency**
(white spots)

66

testine and the ring finger to the kidney. The little finger relates to the heart.

A white spot on the ring finger indicates calcium deposits in the kidney. If the spot is on the middle finger, there is unabsorbed calcium in the intestine. If the white spot is on the index finger, it indicates calcium deposits in the lungs.

Diagram 10
Eye Diagnosis

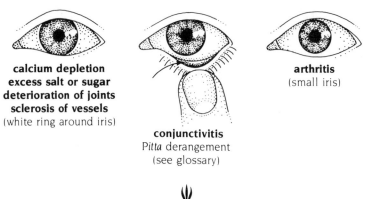

| VATA | PITTA | KAPHA |

Vata eyes are small and nervous, with drooping eyelids and dry, scanty lashes. The white of the eye is muddy, while the iris is dark, grey-brown or black. *Pitta* eyes are moderate in size, sharp, lustrous and sensitive to light. The lashes are scanty and oily while the iris is red or yellowish. *Kapha* eyes are large, beautiful and moist, with long, thick, oily lashes. The white of the eye is very white, while the iris is pale, blue or black.

calcium depletion
excess salt or sugar
deterioration of joints
sclerosis of vessels
(white ring around iris)

conjunctivitis
Pitta derangement
(see glossary)

arthritis
(small iris)

EYE DIAGNOSIS

Eyes that are small and blink frequently show a predominance of *vata* in the body. Excessive blinking shows deep-seated nervousness and anxiety or fear. A drooping upper eyelid indicates a sense of insecurity, fear or lack of confidence, deranged *vata*.

Big, beautiful and attractive eyes indicate a *kapha* constitution.

Pitta eyes are lustrous and sensitive to light, with reddened whites and have a tendency to be nearsighted. According to Ayurveda, the eyes derive their energy from the basic fire element. The fiery energy in the retina results in sensitivity to light. Thus, people of *pitta* constitution, having an abundance of fire in the body, often have eyes that are hypersensitive to light.

If the eyes are prominent, there is a dysfunction of the thyroid gland. If the conjunctiva is pale, anemia is present; if it is yellow, the liver is weak.

One should also examine the color, size and shape of the iris. A small iris indicates weak joints. If there is a white ring around the iris, there is excessive intake of salt or sugar. In the middle-aged, this also may be a sign of bodily stress. If the white ring is very prominent and very white (especially in the middle-aged), this indicates degeneration in the joints. The joints will pop and crack and arthritis and joint pain are likely. Brownish-black spots in the iris indicate unabsorbed iron in the intestine.

In addition to the diagnostic techniques mentioned in the previous pages, Ayurveda also employs other means of clinical examination, namely, palpation, percussion, auscultation and inquiry. Additionally, there are examinations of the heart, liver, spleen, kidney, urine, stool, sputum, sweat, speech and physiognomy.

CHAPTER VII
Treatment

A ll Ayurvedic treatment attempts to establish a balance between the bodily humors, *vata-pitta-kapha*. As discussed in the fourth chapter, disease results when these three are out of balance.

According to Ayurvedic teaching, the initiation of any form of treatment (whether it be medication, acupuncture, chiropractic, massage, allopathy or any other) without first eliminating the toxins in the system that are responsible for the disease, will only push these poisons deeper into the tissues. Symptomatic relief of the disease process may result from superficial treatment. However, the fundamental cause of the illness will not be affected and the problem will therefore manifest again in the same or another form.

There are two types of Ayurvedic treatment: elimination of toxins and neutralization of toxins. These treatments may be applied on both the physical and emotional levels.

EMOTIONAL RELEASE

Let us first deal with the emotional or psychological factors. Anger, fear, anxiety, nervousness, jealousy, possessiveness and greed are common human emotions. Yet most people learn in childhood not to express these negative emotions. As a result, one begins at an early age to repress the natural expressions of these feelings. The science of Ayurveda teaches that the individual must release these emotions which, if they remain repressed, will cause imbalances resulting in disease-causing toxins.

The Ayurvedic technique for dealing with negativity is: observation and release. For example, when anger appears, one should be completely aware of it; watch this feeling as it unfolds from beginning to end. From this observation, one can learn about the nature of the anger and then let the anger go, release it. All negative emotions may be dealt with in this way. Ayurveda teaches that through awareness all negative emotions can be released.

Fear is associated with *vata*; anger with *pitta*; and greed, envy and possessiveness with *kapha*. If one represses fear, the kidneys will be disturbed; anger, the liver; greed and possessiveness, the heart and spleen.

THE PANCHA KARMA

For numerous ailments such as excess mucus in the chest, bile in the intestines, *kapha* in the stomach or gas accumulation in the large intestine, physical elimination may be used. For such treatment, Ayurveda suggests *pancha karma*. These processes are cleansing to the body, mind and emotions. *Pancha* means "five" and *karma* means "actions" or "process". The five basic processes are: vomiting; purgatives or laxatives; medicated enemas; nasal administration of medication and purification of the blood.

THERAPEUTIC VOMITING (Vaman)

When there is congestion in the lungs causing repeated attacks of bronchitis, cough, cold or asthma, the Ayurvedic treatment is therapeutic vomiting (*vamana*), to eliminate the mucus-causing excess *kapha*. First, three or four glasses of licorice or calamus root tea are administered; then vomiting is stimulated by rubbing the tongue, which releases emotions. Or, in the morning before brushing the teeth, one may take two glasses of salt water, which will aggravate *kapha*. Then rub the tongue to induce vomiting. Once the mucus is released, the patient will feel instantly relieved. Congestion, wheezing and breathlessness will disappear and the sinuses will become clear.

Therapeutic vomiting is also indicated for skin diseases, chronic asthma, diabetes, chronic cold, lymphatic obstruction, chronic indigestion, edema (swelling), epilepsy (between attacks), chronic sinus problems and repeated attacks of tonsillitis.

PURGATIVES (Virechan)

When much bile is secreted and accumulated in the gall-bladder, liver or intestines, an allergic rash or skin inflammation,

Chart 5
Emesis Therapy (Vaman)
Elimination through the Upper Pathways

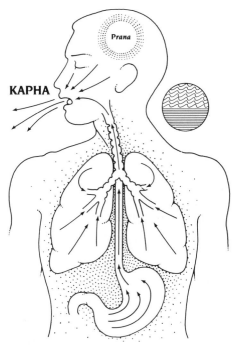

Vaman is the cleansing of *Kapha* and the elimination of mucus & congestion.

Pre-Emesis Measures: Oil massage and fomentation are administered on the night before the day of *Vaman*. One to three days prior to *Vaman*, the person should drink one cup of oil two to three times a day until the stool becomes oily, or he feels nauseated. He should also eat a *Kaphagenic* diet to aggravate *Kapha* in the system. *Vaman* should be given in the morning (*Kapha* time). The person should eat Basmati rice and yogurt with much salt early in the morning, which will further aggravate *Kapha* in the stomach. The application of heat to the chest and back will liquify the *Kapha*. The person should sit calmly on a knee-high chair, and drink a concoction of licorice and honey, or calamus root tea. This emesis preparation is measured and recorded before being drunk, so that at a later time the amount of vomitis from the decoction can be determined. After drinking the decoction, the person should feel nauseated. He should then rub the tongue to induce vomiting, continuing until bile comes out in the vomitis. The degree of success in this treatment is determined by: 1) the

71

number of vomitings (8 is maximum, 6 medium, 4 minimum), and 2) the quantity of vomitus (1 quart maximum, 1½ pints medium, 1 pint minimum).

Post-Emesis Measures: Resting, fasting, smoking medicated cigarettes, and not suppressing natural urges, i.e. urination, defecation, gas, sneezing, coughing

Indications: Cough, cold, symptoms of asthma, *Kapha* fever, nausea, loss of appetite, anemia, bleeding through lower channels, poisoning, skin diseases, diabetes, lymphatic obstruction, chronic indigestion, edema (swelling), epilepsy, chronic sinus problems, repeated attacks of tonsillitis

Contra-indications: Childhood, old age, debility, hunger, heart disease, cavities in the lungs, bleeding of upper channels, menstruation, pregnancy, emaciation, grief, obesity

Emetics (Substances): Licorice, calamus, salt, cardamom, nux vomica

Chart 6
Purgation Therapy (*Virechan*)
Elimination through the Lower Pathways

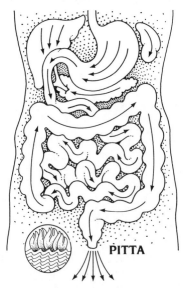

PITTA

Virechan is the cleansing of *Pitta* and the purification of blood toxins. It can be given three days after *Vaman* therapy. If *Vaman* therapy is not indicated, it can be administered directly. To prepare for *Virechan* therapy, oil and fomentation must be applied to the rectum and abdomen respectively. *Virechan* cleanses the sweat glands, small intestine, colon, kidneys,

72

stomach, liver and spleen.

Indications: Skin diseases, chronic fever, piles, abdominal tumours, worms, gout, jaundice

Possible Contra-Indications: Childhood, old age, debility, acute fever, low *Agni*, indigestion, bleeding from lower channels, cavities in lungs, diarrhea, foreign body in stomach, immediately after *Vaman*, emaciation, ulcerative colitis, prolapsed rectum

Virechan Substances: Senna, prune, bran, flaxseed husk, dandelion root, pysllium seed, cow's milk, salt, castor oil, raisins, mango juice

such as acne or dermatitis, as well as chronic fever, ascites, biliary vomiting or jaundice may result. The Ayurvedic treatment for this condition is administration of purgatives or laxatives (*virechan*). A number of fine herbs grown in the United States can be used for this treatment. For example, senna leaf tea is a mild laxative. However, in people of *vata* constitution, this tea might create griping pain, since its action aggravates peristaltic movement in the large intestine.

An effective laxative for *vata* or *pitta* constitutions is a glass of hot milk to which two teaspoons of *ghee* have been added. (The preparation of *ghee* is described in Appendix C - Recipes.) This laxative, taken at bedtime will help to relieve the excess *pitta* causing the bile disturbance in the body. In fact, purgatives can completely cure the problem of excessive *pitta*.

When purgatives are used, it is important to check the diet. The patient should not eat foods that will aggravate the predominant humor or cause the three humors to become unbalanced. (For more details on diet, see Chapter VIII.)

Purgatives should not be given to persons with low *agni*, acute fever, diarrhea, severe constipation or bleeding from the rectum or the lung cavities. Nor should they be administered when a foreign body is present in the stomach, after enema, or in cases of emaciation, weakness or prolapsed rectum.

ENEMA (Basti)

Ayurvedic enema treatment (*basti*) involves introduction into the

Chart 7
Enema Therapy (Basti)
Elimination and Medication through the Lower Pathways

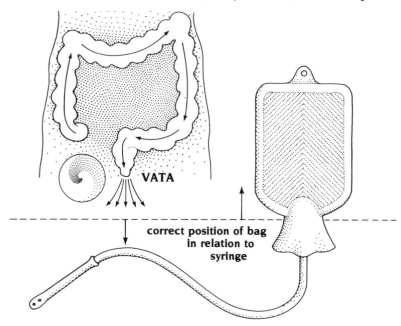

Vata is the main etiological factor in the manifestation of disease. Vata is responsible for the retention or elimination of feces, urine, bile and other excretas.

Vata is mainly located in the colon. Bones are also the site of Vata. Hence, the medication administered rectally works up to the Asthi Dhatu. The mucus membrane of the colon is related to the outer covering of the bones (periosteum), which nourishes the bones. Therefore, any medication given rectally goes into the deeper tissues, like bones, and corrects Vata disorders.

Types of Enemas: 1) Oil Enema — ½ to 1 cup of warm sesame oil (for chronic constipation), 2) Decoction Enema — ½ cup of gotu kola or comfrey decoction (see licorice decoction listed under licorice *ghee* in recipe section) with ½ cup of warm sesame oil, 3) Nutrition Enema - 1 cup of warm milk, 1 cup of meat broth or 1 cup of bone marrow soup

Indications: Constipation, distention, low back ache, gout, rheumatism, sciatica, arthritis, nervous disorders, Vata headache, emaciation, muscular atrophy

Contra-Indications: 1) Oil Enema - Diabetes, obesity, indigestion, low *agni*, enlarged spleen, unconsciousness, 2) Decoction Enema - Debility, hiccough, hemorrhoids, inflammation of anus, diarrhea, pregnancy, ascites, diabetes, 3) Nutrition Enema - Diabetes, obesity, lymphatic obstruction, ascites.

rectum of medicinals such as sesame oil, calamus oil or herbal decoctions in a liquid medium. Medicated enema is the complete treatment for *vata* disorders. It alleviates constipation, distention, chronic fever, the common cold, sexual disorders, kidney stones, heart pain, vomiting, backache, neck pain and hyperacidity. Many *vata* disorders such as sciatica, arthritis, rheumatism and gout also are treated with enemas. V*ata* is a very active principle in pathogenesis, and there are at least eighty different *vata*-related disorders. B*asti* is a complete treatment for eighty percent of these diseases.

Medicated enemas should not be given if the patient is suffering from diarrhea or bleeding from the rectum. An oil enema should not be given to persons having chronic indigestion, cough, breathlessness, diarrhea, diabetes or severe anemia; nor to the aged or children below seven years of age. Decoction enemas (herbs boiled in water) should not be given for acute fever, diarrhea, cold, paralysis, heart pain, severe pain in the abdomen or emaciation. Oil or decoction enemas should be retained for a minimum of thirty minutes; however, it is best to retain longer if possible.

NASAL ADMINISTRATION (Nasya)

The nasal administration of medication is called *nasya*. An excess of bodily humors accumulated in the throat, nose, sinus or head is elimininated by means of the nearest possible opening. The nose is the door to the brain and to consciousness: *prana* or life energy, enters the body through breath taken in through the nose. P*rana* maintains sensory and motor functions. Nasal administration of medication helps to correct the disorders of *prana* affecting the higher cerebral, sensory and motor functions.

Nasal administration is indicated for dryness of the nose, sinus congestion, hoarseness, migraine headache, convulsions and certain eye and ear problems. In general, nasal medication should not be administered after a bath, food, sex or drinking alcohol, nor should it be applied during pregnancy or menstruation.

Breathing also can be improved through nasal massage. For this treatment, the little finger is dipped into *ghee* and inserted into the nose. The inner walls of the nose are slowly massaged, going as deeply as possible. This treatment will help to open the emotions. (Nose tissue is tender and for this application the fingernail must be kept short to avoid injuring the delicate mucus membranes.) Since most people have deviated nasal septums, one side

Chart 8
Nasal Administration (Nasya)
The Nose Is the Door to the Brain and Consciousness

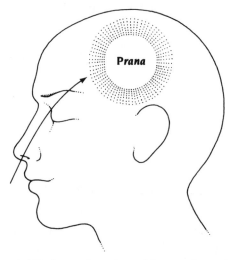

Prana

Types of Nasya: 1) Virechana (cleansing with use of powders or herbs), 2) Nutritional Nasya (for Vata), 3) Sedative Nasya, 4) Nasya Decoctions, 5) Ghee or Oil Nasya, 6) Nasal Massage

Administration of Powder: A dry powder of gotu kola is blown into the nose with a tube. It is used in Kapha disorders, i.e. headache, heaviness in the head, cold, running of nose, sticky eyes, hoarseness due to sticky Kapha, sinusitis, cervical lymphadenitis, tumours, worms, skin diseases, epilepsy, drowsiness, Parkinsonism, chronic rhinitis, attachment, greed, lust.

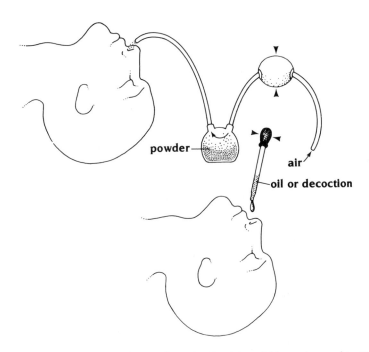

powder

air

oil or decoction

Nutritional Nasya: Use ghee, oils, salt. Nutritional Nasya is used in Vata disorders, i.e. migraine headache, dryness of voice, dry nose, nervousness, anxiety, fear, dizziness, emptiness, negativity, ptosis, bursitis, stiffness in the neck, cervical spondylosis, dry sinuses, loss of sense of smell.

Sedative Nasya: Use aloe vera juice, warm milk, juice of asparagus root, gotu kola juice. Sedative Nasya is used only in Pitta disorders, i.e. hairfall, conjunctivitis, ringing in the ear.

Oil Nasya: Decoctions and oils together are used in Vata, Pitta or Kapha disorders.

Nasal Massage: Dip the clean little finger into the appropriate oil and insert into each nostril as deeply as possible. The nasal passage is then lubricated through this gentle massage. Nasal massage helps to relax the deeper tissues and can be done every day or any time one is under stress.

As shown in the diagram, the person should lie on the table with the head down and the nose facing up. Put 5 drops of oil or decoction as needed into each nostril. Lie in this position for one minute or more.

Contra-Indications: Pregnancy, menstruation; after sex, bathing, eating, or drinking alcohol

Substances Used in Nasya: Calamus powder, gotu kola, onion, garlic, black pepper, cayenne, ginger, *ghee* oil decoctions.

of the nose will be easier to penetrate and massage than the other. The finger should not be inserted forcibly. The massage should proceed by slow penetration, the finger moving first in a clockwise, then in a counterclockwise direction. By this means, the emotions that are blocked in the respiratory tract will be released. One may use this treatment each morning and evening. In this way, breathing patterns will change as the emotions are released and the eyesight also will improve.

BLOOD-LETTING (Rakta Moksha)

Toxins that are absorbed into the bloodstream through the gastrointestinal tract circulate throughout the body. They may manifest under the skin or in the joint-spaces, creating disease. In such cases, elimination of toxins and purification of the blood is necessary.

For repeated attacks of skin disorders such as urticaria, rash, eczema, acne, scabies, leucoderma, chronic itching and hives, blood-letting (rakta moksha) is indicated. It also is effective in cases of enlarged liver and spleen, and for gout.

Pitta is manifested in the waste products of the blood, so in many pitta disorders, such as rash and acne, the toxins are circulated in the blood system. Thus, for many pitta ailments, extracting a small amount of blood from the vein relieves the tension created by the toxins in the blood.*

Blood-letting also stimulates antitoxic substances in the blood stream which helps develop the immune mechanism in the blood system. Thus, the toxins are neutralized enabling radical cures of many blood and bone disorders.

Blood-letting also is contra-indicated in cases of anemia, edema and weakness. This treatment is not recommended for young children or the aged.

Some subtances such as excess sugar, salt, yogurt and sour-tasting foods are toxic to the blood. In certain blood disorders, to keep the blood pure, these substances should be avoided.

---

*This procedure should be administered only by a physician.

Burdock root tea

Burdock root tea is the best blood-purifier. For blood-carried disorders such as allergy, rash or acne the patient should take a milk laxative and the next evening begin burdock root tea therapy. The tea is made from one teaspoon of powder in one cup of hot water. If taken every night, the action of the herb will begin to purify the blood. Other blood-purifying herbs are saffron, sandalwood powder, turmeric and calamus root powder. Pomegranate juice, orange juice and asparagus root are also beneficial for blood ailments. These may be used after blood-letting has been performed.

PALLIATION

Following treatment to eliminate the most serious toxins, the process of palliation (*shamana*) is employed. Palliation involves neutralizing the toxins by enkindling *agni* and stimulating the digestion through fasting. Toxins also may be neutralized by internal use of hot, pungent herbs such as ginger and black pepper. Sustained hunger and thirst, exercise, sunbathing and sitting in the fresh air are other means of neutralizing toxins.

R   neutralize toxins

CHAPTER VIII
Diet

Ayurveda teaches that each individual has the power to heal himself. Thus, this science of life offers everyone the freedom to recover health by understanding the body and its needs.

Fundamental to the individual's ability to remain healthy, according to Ayurveda, are the maintenance of a sound diet and a stable, healthy routine. Also important are the pursuit of traditional practices such as yoga and breathing exercises; and an understanding of the spiritual practices that can create harmony and happiness.

Diet should be chosen to suit the individual constitution. If one understands the constitution and its relationship to the qualities of various foods, then it is possible to select a proper diet. One needs to take into account the taste of the food (sweet, sour, salty, pungent, bitter or astringent) and also whether it is heavy or light, hot- or cold-producing, oily or dry, liquid or solid. The seasons of the year must also be considered in choosing diet.

The accompanying table provides a list of the foods that are helpful or harmful for each constitution. The up-pointing arrows next to each food category on the chart indicate that these substances aggravate the corresponding factor. The down-pointing arrows indicate foods that decrease the humor such foods being good for the individual of that particular constitution. For instance, dry fruits, apples, melons, potatoes, tomatoes, eggplant, ice cream, beef, peas and green salad aggravate *vata*. Thus, they should not be taken in excess by a person of *vata* constitution. Conversely, sweet fruits, avocados, coconut, brown rice, red cabbage, bananas, grapes, cherries and oranges are beneficial for people of *vata* constitution.

Increase of the *pitta dosha* will be caused by spicy foods, peanut butter, sour fruits, bananas, papayas, tomatoes and garlic. Foods that inhibit *pitta* are: mangoes, oranges, pears, plums, sprouts, green salad, sunflower seeds, asparagus and mushrooms.

Bananas, melons, coconut, dates, papayas, pineapples and dairy products increase *kapha*. However, dry fruits, pomegranates, cranberries, basmati rice, sprouts and chicken are beneficial for people of *kapha* constitution.

During summer, when the temperature is high, people tend to perspire excessively. *Pitta* predominates at that time of year. It is not good to eat hot, spicy or pungent foods then because they will aggravate *pitta*. During autumn, when the wind is high and dry, more *vata* is present in the atmosphere. At this time, one should avoid dry fruits, high protein foods and other foods that increase *vata*. Winter is the season of *kapha*; it brings cold and snow. During this period one should avoid cold drinks, ice cream, cheese and yogurt. Such foods will increase *kapha*.

When considering diet, the quality and freshness of food are important factors. There also are certain foods that are incompatible when eaten together, such as fish and milk, meat and milk, yogurt and beef, and sour fruits and milk. In addition, most melons should be eaten alone. In combination with other foods, they create clogging and may prevent absorption by the intestines. These effects could cause an imbalance in the *tridosha*. Toxins result when these incompatible foods are ingested together.

The intake of food should be regulated by the condition of the *agni*, the digestive fire in the body. Do not eat unless you feel hungry and do not drink unless you are thirsty. Do not eat when you feel thirsty and do not drink when you feel hungry. If you feel hungry, it means your digestive fire is enkindled. If you drink at this time, the liquid will dissolve the digestive enzymes and the *agni* will be reduced.

It is food that nourishes the body, mind and consciousness. How you eat is very important. While eating, one should sit straight and avoid distractions such as television, conversation or reading. Focus your mind upon and be aware of the taste of the food. Chew with love and compassion and you will clearly experience the taste.

Taste does not originate in food, it originates in the experience of the one who eats. If your *agni* is impaired, you will not taste the

Table 5

Food Guidelines for Basic Constitutional Types

NOTE: Guidelines provided in this table are general. Specific adjustments for individual requirements may need to be made. e.g. food allergies, strength of agni, season of the year, and degree of dosha predominance or aggravation. _Autumn/Spring_ _Summer_ _Winter_

▲ Aggravates Dosha
▼ Balances Dosha

	VATA		PITTA		KAPHA	
	NO ▲	YES ▼	NO ▲	YES ▼	NO ▲	YES ▼
FRUITS	Dried Fruits	Sweet Fruits	Sour Fruits	Sweet Fruits	Sweet & Sour	Apples
	Apples	Apricots	Apricots	Apples	Fruits	Apricots
	Cranberries	Avocado	Berries	Avocado	Avocado	Berries
	Pears	Bananas	Bananas	Coconut	Bananas	Cherries
	Persimmon	Berries	Cherries	Figs	Coconut	Cranberries
	Pomegranate	Cherries	Cranberries	Grapes (dark)	Figs (fresh)	Figs (dry)
	Watermelon	Coconut	Grapefruit	Mango	Grapefruit	Mango
		Figs (fresh)	Grapes (green)	Melons	Grapes	Peaches
		Grapefruit	Lemons	Oranges (sweet)	Lemons	Pears
		Grapes	Oranges (sour)	Pears	Melons	Persimmon
		Lemons	Papaya	Pineapples (sweet)	Oranges	Pomegranate
		Mango	Peaches	Plums (sweet)	Papaya	Prunes
		Melons (sweet)	Pineapples (sour)	Pomegranate	Pineapples	Raisins
		Oranges	Persimmon	Prunes	Plums	
		Papaya	Plums (sour)	Raisins		
		Peaches				
		Pineapples				
		Plums				
VEGETABLES	Raw Vegetables	Cooked	Pungent	Sweet & Bitter	Sweet & Juicy	Pungent & Bitter
	Broccoli	Vegetables	Vegetables	Vegetables	Vegetables	Vegetables
	Brussels Sprouts	Asparagus	Beets	Asparagus	Cucumber	Asparagus
	Cabbage	Beets	Carrots	Broccoli	Potatoes (sweet)	Beets
	Cauliflower	Carrots	Eggplant	Brussels Sprouts	Tomatoes	Broccoli

82

Celery	Cucumber	Garlic	Cabbage	Zucchini	Brussels Sprouts
Eggplant	Garlic	Onions	Cucumber		Cabbage
Leafy Greens*	Green Beans	Peppers (hot)	Cauliflower		Carrots
Lettuce*	Okra (cooked)	Radishes	Celery		Cauliflower
Mushrooms	Onion (cooked)	Spinach	Green Beans		Celery
Onions (raw)	Potato (sweet)	Tomatoes	Leafy Greens		Eggplant
Parsley*	Radishes		Lettuce		Garlic
Peas	Zucchini		Mushrooms		Leafy Greens
Peppers			Okra		Lettuce
Potatoes (white)			Peas		Mushrooms
Spinach*			Parsley		Okra
Sprouts*			Peppers (green)		Onions
Tomatoes			Potatoes		Parsley
			Sprouts		Peas
			Zucchini		Peppers
					Potatoes (white)
					Radishes
					Spinach
					Sprouts

These Vegetables are OK in moderation. with oil dressing.

GRAINS					
Barley	Oats (cooked)	Buckwheat	Barley	Oats (cooked)	Barley
Buckwheat	Rice	Corn	Oats (cooked)	Rice (brown)	Corn
Corn	Wheat	Millet	Rice (basmati)	Rice (white)	Millet
Millet		Oats (dry)	Rice (white)	Wheat	Oats (dry)
Oats (dry)		Rice (brown)	Wheat		Rice (basmati, small amount)
Rye		Rye			Rye

ANIMAL FOODS					
Lamb	Beef	Beef	Chicken or Turkey (white meat)	Beef	Chicken or Turkey (dark meat)
Pork	Chicken or Turkey (white meat)	Eggs (yolk)	Eggs (white)	Lamb	Eggs (not fried scrambled)
Rabbit	Eggs (fried or scrambled)	Lamb	Rabbit	Pork	Rabbit
Venison		Pork		Seafood	
		Seafood			

83

Table 5, continued

	VATA NO ▲	VATA YES ▼	PITTA NO ▲	PITTA YES ▼	KAPHA NO ▲	KAPHA YES ▼
ANIMAL FOODS *continued*		Seafood		Shrimp (small amount) Venison		Shrimp Venison
LEGUMES	No Legumes except Mung Beans, Tofu, Black & Red Lentils		All Legumes OK except Lentils		All Legumes are Good except Kidney Beans, Soy-Beans, Black Lentils & Mung Beans	
NUTS		All Nuts are OK in Small Quantities	No Nuts except Coconut		No Nuts at All	
SEEDS		All Seeds are OK (in moderation)	No Seeds except Sunflower & Pumpkin		No Seeds except Sunflower & Pumpkin	
SWEETENERS		All Sweeteners are OK except White Sugar	All Sweeteners are OK except Molasses & Honey		No Sweeteners except Raw Honey	
CONDIMENTS		All Spices are Good	No Spices except Coriander, Cinnamon, Cardamom, Fennel, Turmeric & a Small Amount of Black Pepper.		All Spices are Good Except Salt	
DAIRY		All Dairy Products are OK (in moderation)	Buttermilk Cheese Sour Cream Yogurt	Butter (unsalted) Cottage Cheese Ghee Milk	No Dairy except Ghee & Goatmilk	
OILS		All Oils are Good	Almond Corn Safflower Sesame	Coconut Olive Sunflower Soy	No Oils except Almond, Corn or Sunflower in Small Amounts	

food properly. The taste of food depends upon *agni*. Spices help to enkindle *agni*, as well as to cleanse the body and to enrich the taste of the food. Each mouthful should be chewed at least thirty-two times before it is swallowed. This practice allows the digestive enzymes in the mouth to do their work properly and, in addition, it gives the stomach time to prepare for the arrival of the masticated food. It is important that one eats at a moderate speed.

How much food you take at one time also is important. One-third of the stomach should be filled with food, one-third with water and one-third with air. The amount of food eaten at a meal should be the equivalent of two handsful of food. If one eats in excess, the stomach will expand and demand additional food. An overeater's stomach expands like a balloon. Overeating also results in the creation of additional toxins in the digestive tract. The food becomes a poison that the body must eliminate through effort. One should eat and drink with discipline and regularity for eating is a meditation. Eating in this way will nourish your body mind and consciousness and will also enhance longevity.

Water plays a vital role in maintaining balance in the body. Water may be taken in the form of fruit juices. Although fruit juice should not be taken during meals, water is necessary at meals. One should sip water while eating. Water taken with meals becomes a nectar that aids digestion. If a quantity of water is drunk after the completion of a meal, the digestive juices will be diluted and digestion hampered. Climate will affect the amount of water the body requires.

If there is indigestion, one should observe a warm-water fast. This practice will aid cleansing and increase *agni*. Cold water will cool down *agni*; therefore, ice cold water is poison to the system and hot water is nectar. The digestion is affected when one drinks a lot of water. Too much water can result in retention and additional body weight.

FASTING

Before a fast is undertaken, consideration must be given to the individual constitution. In the West, people sometimes observe fasts for ten, fifteen, twenty or more days without considering their constitutions. This lack of understanding of constitutional requirements may have detrimental effects.

A person of *vata* constitution should not observe a fast for more than three days. Not eating increases lightness in the body and *vata* (bodily air) is also light. So, the *vata* element becomes impaired if a fast is continued too long and this impaired element will create fear, anxiety, nervousness, and weakness.

The same restriction on length of fasting holds for individuals of *pitta* constitution. A fast of more than four days will aggravate *pitta*, increasing the fire element in the body. This increased *pitta* will cause psycho/physical reactions of anger, hate and dizziness.

People with *kapha* constitutions, however, may observe prolonged fasts. They will feel a pleasant sensation of increased lightness, greater awareness and an opening of consciousness. Clarity and understanding will improve.

If a juice fast is undertaken, it is important to remember that grape juice is good for the *vata* constitution; pomegranate juice for the *pitta* constitution; and apple juice for the *kapha* constitution. Each day of the fast, drink about one and one-half quarts of the juice diluted with water.

The digestive system is resting during a fast. It is important not to place strain on the *agni*, the digestive fire, during this time. During fasting, the digestive fire becomes enkindled and, since there is no food to digest, *agni slowly burns away the long-existing toxins in the intestines*.

Ayurveda teaches that during a fast certain herbs such as ginger, black pepper, cayenne pepper and curry, which have medicinal value because of their hot, spicy attributes, may be used to help neutralize toxins in the system. If these herbs are taken in the form of tea, they will help enkindle *agni* which will burn away toxins.

When one is observing a fast, physical strength and stamina should be watched. If it becomes noticeably less, the fast should be discontinued.

Fasting is recommended when there is fever, cold, constipation or arthritic pain. If there are toxins, or if *ama* exists in the large intestine, fasting is indicated.

For the normal, healthy individual, a warm water fast (one to two quarts per day) is advisable at least one day a week. This practice allows the digestive system to rest.

VITAMINS

In the West, taking vitamins is regarded as a means to create or maintain good health. Physicians and health-professionals prescribe vitamins routinely to their patients and such practices as taking massive doses of vitamin C to prevent colds are common. However, if the individual constitution is not considered, such doses of vitamins may create imbalances in the *dosha*. The human body has a capacity to generate the vitamins it needs and dependence upon external vitamins, without consideration of the individual constitution and condition of *agni*, may create an excess of vitamins in the body (hypervitaminosis).

Many people who regularly take vitamins and minerals to supplement their diets continue to suffer from the same deficiencies for which they are taking supplements because they are unable to properly digest, assimilate and absorb these natural and synthetic vitamins.

CHAPTER IX

Taste

The element of water is the basis for the sensory experience of taste. The tongue must be wet in order to taste a substance. Try drying your tongue and then putting a small amount of sugar or pepper on it. You will not be able to taste it. A wet tongue is necessary for the perception of taste.

There are six tastes: sweet, sour, salty, pungent. bitter and astringent. These six basic tastes are derived from the five elements. The sweet taste contains Earth and Water elements; sour, Earth and Fire; and salty, Water and Fire. The pungent taste contains Fire and Air; bitter, Air and Ether; and astringent, Air and Earth.

People of *vata* constitution should avoid bitter, pungent and astringent substances in excess which increase air and have a tendency to cause gas. Substances containing sweet, sour and salty tastes are good for individuals of *vata* constitutions.

People of *pitta* constitution should avoid sour, salty and pungent substances which aggravate bodily fire. However, sweet , bitter and astringent tastes are beneficial for individuals of *pitta* constitution.

Kapha individuals should avoid foods containing sweet, sour and salty tastes for they increase bodily water. They should choose food of pungent, bitter and astringent tastes.

RASA, VIRYA AND VIPAK

Ayurvedic pharmacology is based upon the concepts of *rasa*, *virya* and *vipak*. These concepts have to do with the subtle phenomena relating to taste and to hot and cold effects of foods. Organic and inorganic substances create different tastes and temperature sensations when they pass through the mouth, stomach, small intestine and large intestine.

When a substance is placed on the tongue, the first experience of that taste is called *rasa*. When a substance is swallowed and then enters the stomach, the hot or cold experience that is felt immediately or later is called *virya*. The *virya* sensation or action, then, has to do with the heating and cooling properties of substances. Food also has a postdigestive effect which is called *vipak*. For instance, most starchy foods become sweet after chewing and digestion, so their postdigestive taste, or *vipak*, is sweet.

The Ayurvedic pharmacology is based upon *rasya*, *virya* and *vipak* of substances. In daily observation it is found that there are numerous other substances which have a specific unexplained action in the body. To acknowledge this action, Charak has used the term *prabhav* which literally means specific action without regard to *rasa*, *virya* and *vipak* or, the exception to the rule. The concept of *rasa*, *virya* and *vipak* is not only applicable to foods and herbs but also to everything including gems, stones, minerals, metals, color and even the mind and emotions. Below is a table which gives the general rules for determining *rasa*, *virya* and *vipak*. Also, an example of *prabhav*, or an exception, is listed for each taste.

Rasa *taste*	Virya *experience*	Vipak *post digestive effect*	Prabhav
Sweet	Cold	Sweet	Honey Hot (*virya*)
Sour	Hot	Sour	Lemon Cold (*virya*)
Salty	Hot	Sweet	Tamari Cold (*virya*)
Pungent	Hot	Pungent	Onion Cold (*virya*)
Bitter	Cold	Pungent	Turmeric Hot (*virya*)
Astringent	Cold	Pungent	Pomegranate Sweet (*vipak*)

Thus, in general, sweet and salty tastes have sweet *vipak*; the sour taste has sour *vipak*, and the pungent, bitter and astringent tastes have pungent *vipak*. Thus, *rasa* and *vipak* are directly related to the tastes of substances, while *virya* is related to their hot and cold effects.

These three directly influence the *tridosha* and also influence nutrition and transformation of the bodily tissues or *dhatus*. These qualities can only be understood through individual experience. The following charts serve as a guideline to assist the reader in understanding *rasa*, *virya* and *vipak* and their properties and actions.

Table 6
Tastes and Their Actions

TASTE	PROPERTY	EXAMPLES	ACTIONS	DISORDERS
Sweet (Earth + Water)	Cooling	Wheat, Rice, Milk, Candy, Sugar, Dates, Licorice Root, Red Clove, Peppermint, Slippery Elm.	Anabolic: Decreases Vata & Pitta. Increases Kapha. Adds Wholesomeness to the Body. Increases Rasa, Water and Ojas. Promotes Strength; Relieves Thirst; Creates a Burning Sensation. Nourishes & Soothes the Body. Is Cold.	Increases Obesity; Causes Excess Sleep, Heaviness, Lethargy, Loss of Appetite, Cough, Diabetes, & Abnormal Growth of Muscles.
Sour (Earth + Fire)	Heating	Yogurt, Cheese, Green Grapes, Lemon, Hibiscus, Rose Hips, Tamarind.	Anabolic: Decreases Vata & Increases Pitta & Kapha. Adds Deliciousness to Food. Stimulates Appetite & Sharpens the Mind. Strengthens the Sense Organs; Causes Secretions & Salivation. Is Light, Hot & Unctuous.	Increases Thirst, Sensitiveness of Teeth, Closure of Eyes. Liquification of Kapha. Toxification of Blood, Edema, Ulcerations, Heartburn & Acidity.
Saline (salty) (Water + Fire)	Heating	Sea Salt, Rock Salt, Kelp.	Anabolic: Decreases Vata & Increases Pitta & Kapha. Helps Digestion. Acts as an Anti-Spasmodic & Laxative. Promotes	Disturbs Blood. Causes Fainting & Heating of the Body. Increases Skin Diseases. Causes Inflammation, Blood Disorders, Peptic

Taste		Herbs	Action	Excess Effects
			Salivation, Nullifies the Effect of All Other Tastes. Retains Water. Heavy. Unctuous. Hot.	Ulcer, Rash, Pimples & Hypertension.
Pungent (Fire + Air)	Heating	Onion, Radish, Chili, Ginger, Garlic, Asafoetida, Cayenne Pepper.	Catabolic; Decreases *Kapha* & *Pitta*. Increases *Vata* & *Pitta*. Keeps the Mouth Clean. Promotes Digestion & Absorption of Food. Purifies the Blood. Cures Skin Disease. Helps to Eliminate Blood Clots. Cleanses the Body. Light. Hot. Unctuous.	Increases Heat, Sweating, Fainting, Creates Burning Sensations in Throat, Stomach & Heart. Can Cause a Peptic Ulcer, Dizziness & Unconsciousness.
Bitter (Air + *Ether*)	Cooling	Dandelion Root, Holy Thistle, Osha, Yellow Dock, Rhubarb, Fresh Turmeric Root, Fennugreek, Gentian Root.	Catabolic; Decreases *Pitta* & *Kapha*. Increases *Vata*. Promotes Other Tastes. Acts as an Antitoxic & Germicidal. Is an Antidote for Fainting, Itching & Burning Sensations in the Body. Is Light & Cold.	Increases Roughness, Emaciation, Dryness. Reduces Bone Marrow & Semen. Can Cause Dizziness & Eventual Unconsciousness.
Astringent (Air + *Earth*)	Cooling	Unripe Banana, Pomegranate, Myrrh, Goldenseal, Turmeric, Alum.	Catabolic; Decreases *Pitta* & *Kapha*. Increases *Vata*. Has a Sedative Action, but Is Constipative. Causes Constriction of Blood Vessels, Coagulation of Blood. Is Dry, Rough, Cold.	Increases Dryness of Mouth, Distension. Constipation. Obstruction of Speech. Too Much Astringent Taste Can Adversely Affect the Heart.

Table 7
Properties and Actions of *Rasa, Virya, Vipak*

SUBSTANCE	TASTE	HEATING OR COOLING	POST-DIGESTIVE EFFECT	PROPERTIES & ACTION ON TRI-DOSHA
Meat				
Beef	Sweet	Heating	Sweet	Heavy, Thick, Increases *Pitta & Kapha*. Reduces *Vata*.
Chicken	Sweet & Astringent	Heating	Pungent	Light. Oily. Strengthening. Moderately OK for *Vata*. *Pitta & Kapha*.
Fish (general)	Sweet	Heating	Sweet	Heavy, Oily, Smooth. Promotes Heat. Increases *Pitta & Kapha*. Reduces *Vata*.
Lamb	Sweet & Astringent	Heating	Sweet	Heavy. Strenthening. Increases *Vata, Pitta & Kapha*.
Pork	Sweet & Astringent	Heating	Sweet	Heavy, Oily, Smooth. Appetizing. Promotes Perspiration. Increases *Vata. Pitta & Kapha*.
Rabbit	Sweet & Astringent	Heating	Pungent	Light. Dry. Rough. Increases *Vata*. Decreases *Pitta & Kapha*.
Dairy				
Butter (unsalted)	Sweet & Astringent	Cooling	Sweet	Oily. Smooth. Reduces Hemorrhoids. Promotes Intestinal Absorption. Increases *Kapha*. Reduces *Vata & Pitta*.
Cheese (unsalted)	Sweet & Sour	Cooling	Sweet	Heavy. Smooth. Increases *Pitta & Kapha*. Decreases *Vata*.

Food	Taste	Energy	Taste	Effects
Cow's Milk	Sweet	Cooling	Sweet	Light, Oily, Smooth. Increases *Kapha*, Decreases *Vata* & *Pitta*.
Eggs	Sweet & Astringent	Heating	Pungent	Oily, Smooth, Heavy. Increases *Pitta* & *Kapha*. Decreases *Vata*.
Ghee	Sweet	Cooling	Sweet	Light, Oily, Smooth. If Taken in Excess, Increases *Kapha*. If Taken Moderately. Good for *Vata*, *Pitta* & *Kapha*. Promotes Digestion. Strengthening.
Goat's Milk	Sweet & Astringent	Cooling	Sweet	Light. Relieves Cough, Fever, Diarrhea. Increases *Vata*. Decreases *Pitta* & *Kapha*.
Mother's Milk	Sweet	Cooling	Sweet	Light, Oily, Smooth. Enhances *Ojas*. Keeps Balance of *Vata Pitta* & *Kapha*.
Yogurt	Sour & Astringent	Heating	Sour	Smooth. Oily. Good for Digestion. Diarrhea. Painful Urination. Increases *Pitta* & *Kapha*. Decreases *Vata*.
Oils				
Castor Oil	Sweet & Bitter	Heating	Pungent	Heavy, Sharp, Oily. Relieves Rheumatic Fever & Constipation.. Increases *Pitta* & *Kapha*. Decreases *Vata*.
Coconut Oil	Sweet	Cooling	Sweet	Relatively Light, Oily, Smooth. Increases *Kapha*, Relieves *Vata* & *Pitta*.
Corn Oil	Sweet	Heating	Sweet	Relatively Light, Oily, Smooth. Increases *Pitta*, Moderately OK for *Vata* & *Kapha*.
Oil (general)	Sweet	Heating	Sweet	Heavy, Oily, Smooth, Strengthening. Increases *Pitta* & *Kapha*. Relieves *Vata*.
Safflower Oil	Sweet & Pungent	Heating	Pungent	Relatively Light, Sharp, Oily. Irritating if Excessive. Increases *Pitta*. Decreases *Vata* & *Kapha*.

Table 7, continued

SUBSTANCE	TASTE	HEATING OR COOLING	POST-DIGESTIVE EFFECT	PROPERTIES & ACTION ON TRI-DOSHA
Oils, *continued*				
Sunflower Oil	Sweet	Cooling	Sweet	Light, Oily, Smooth, Strengthening. Good for *Vata, Pitta & Kapha.*
White Mustard Oil	Pungent	Heating	Pungent	Light, Sharp, Oily, Relieves Arthritis & Muscle Sprain When Applied Externally with Castor Oil. Increases *Pitta.* Decreases *Vata & Kapha.*
Sesame Oil	Sweet, Bitter & Astringent	Heating	Sweet	Heavy, Oily, Smooth. Increases *Pitta.* Decreases *Vata.* Moderately OK for *Kapha.*
Sweeteners				
Honey (general)	Sweet & Astringent	Heating	Sweet	Dry, Rough, Heavy, Cuts Mucus. Slightly Increases *Pitta.* Decreases *Vata & Kapha.*
Maple Syrup	Sweet & Bitter	Cooling	Sweet	Smooth, Unctuous. May increase *Kapha* If Taken in Excess, Relieves *Vata & Pitta.*
Raw Cane Sugar	Sweet	Cooling	Sweet	Heavy, Smooth, Oily. Increases Fat. Increases *Kapha.* Relieves *Vata & Pitta.*
Legumes				
Black Lentil	Sweet	Heating	Sweet	Strengthening. Increases *Pitta & Kapha.* Decreases *Vata.*
Garbanzos	Sweet & Astringent	Cooling	Sweet	Heavy, Dry, Rough, Very Dehydrating. Produces Gas. Increases *Vata.* Relieves *Pitta & Kapha.*

94

Food	Rasa	Virya	Vipaka	Qualities & Effects
Kidney Beans	Sweet & Astringent	Cooling	Sweet	Dry, Rough, Heavy, Laxative. Increases *Vata & Kapha*. Decreases *Pitta*.
Lentils (general)	Sweet & Astringent	Cooling	Sweet	Dry, Rough, Heavy, Dehydrating. Should Be Taken in Small Quantities. Increases *Vata & Kapha*. Decreases *Pitta*.
Mung Beans	Sweet & Astringent	Cooling	Sweet	Light, Soft. Increases *Kapha*. Decreases *Vata & Pitta*.
Red Lentil	Sweet & Astringent	Heating	Sweet	Easy to Digest. Increases *Pitta*. Relieves *Vata & Kapha*.
Soy Beans	Sweet & Astringent	Cooling	Sweet	Heavy, Oily, Smooth. Laxative. Increases *Vata & Kapha*. Decreases *Pitta*. Tofu is OK for *Vata & Pitta*. Moderately OK for *Kapha*.

Vegetables

Food	Rasa	Virya	Vipaka	Qualities & Effects
Beet	Sweet	Heating	Sweet	Heavy, Smooth. Relieves Anemia. May Increase *Pitta & Kapha* When Taken in Excess. Decreases *Vata*.
Broccoli	Sweet & Astringent	Cooling	Pungent	Rough, Dry. Increases *Vata*, Decreases *Pitta & Kapha*.
Cabbage	Sweet & Astringent	Cooling	Pungent	Rough, Dry. Increases *Vata*, Decreases *Pitta & Kapha*.
Carrot	Sweet, Bitter & Astringent	Cooling	Pungent	Heavy, Reduces Hemorrhoids. Increases *Pitta* if Taken in Excess. Reduces *Vata & Kapha*.
Cauliflower	Astringent	Cooling	Pungent	Rough, Dry. Increases *Vata*, Decreases *Pitta & Kapha*.
Celery	Astringent	Cooling	Pungent	Rough, Dry, Light. Light to Digest, Promotes Gas. Increases *Vata*. Relieves *Pitta & Kapha*.

Table 7, continued

SUBSTANCE	TASTE	HEATING OR COOLING	POST-DIGESTIVE EFFECT	PROPERTIES & ACTION ON TRI-DOSHA
Vegetables, continued				
Cucumber	Sweet & Astringent	Cooling	Sweet	Heavy. Increases *Kapha*. Relieves *Vata* & *Pitta*.
Lettuce (leafy)	Astringent	Cooling	Pungent	Light. Rough. Watery. Easy to Digest. Creates Lightness in the Body. Promotes Gas if Taken in Excess. Increases *Vata*. Relieves *Pitta* & *Kapha*.
Okra	Sweet & Astringent	Cooling	Pungent	Rough. Slimy. OK for *Vata*, *Pitta* & *Kapha*.
Onion (raw)	Pungent	Heating	Pungent	Heavy. Stimulates Sex. Appetizing. Strengthening. Relieves Fever When Applied Externally. Increases *Vata* & *Pitta*. Relieves *Kapha*.
Potato (white)	Sweet, Salty & Astringent	Cooling	Sweet	Dry, Rough, Light. Increases *Vata*. Decreases *Pitta* & *Kapha*.
Radish	Pungent	Heating	Pungent	Relieves Gas. Promotes Digestion. May Increase *Pitta*. Decreases *Vata* & *Kapha*.
Spinach	Astringent	Cooling	Pungent	Rough. Dry. Increases *Vata* & *Pitta*. Decreases *Kapha*.
Sprouts (general)	Mildly Astringent	Cooling	Sweet	Light to Digest. May Aggravate *Vata* if Taken in Excess. Good for *Pitta* & *Kapha*.
Tomato	Sweet & Sour	Heating	Sour	Light. Moist. Increases *Vata*, *Pitta* & *Kapha*.
Zucchini	Sweet & Astringent	Cooling	Pungent	Wet. Light. May Increase *Kapha*. OK for *Vata*. Relieves *Pitta*.

Fruits

Apple	Sweet & Astringent	Cooling	Sweet	Light, Rough. Increases *Vata*. Decreases *Pitta*. OK for *Kapha* in small quantities.
Banana	Sweet & Astringent	Cooling	Sour	Smooth, Heavy. Laxative if Taken in Excess. Increases *Pitta & Kapha*. Decreases *Vata*.
Coconut	Sweet	Cooling	Sweet	Oily, Smooth, Strengthening. Increases *Kapha* if Taken in Excess. Relieves *Vata & Pitta*.
Figs (ripe)	Sweet & Astringent	Cooling	Sweet	Heavy, Nourishing. Delays Digestion. Increases *Kapha*. Relieves *Vata & Pitta*.
Grapes (purple)	Sweet, Sour & Astringent	Cooling	Sweet	Smooth, Watery, Strengthening, Laxative. Increases *Kapha*. Decreases *Vata & Pitta*.
Melons (general)	Sweet	Cooling	Sweet	Heavy, Watery. Increases *Kapha*. Relieves *Vata & Pitta*. Watermelon Increases *Vata*.
Orange	Sweet & Sour	Heating	Sweet	Heavy. Promotes Appetite. Difficult to Digest. Increases *Pitta & Kapha*. Decreases *Vata*.
Peaches	Sweet & Astringent	Heating	Sweet	Heavy, Watery. Increases *Pitta & Kapha*. Decreases *Vata*.
Pears	Sweet & Astringent	Cooling	Sweet	Heavy, Dry, Rough. Increases *Vata*. Reduces *Pitta & Kapha*.
Plums (sweet)	Sweet & Astringent	Heating	Sweet	Heavy, Watery. Increases *Pitta & Kapha*. Decreases *Vata*.
Pomegranate	Sweet, Sour & Astringent	Cooling	Sweet	Smooth, Oily, Stimulates Digestion. Helps to Form Red Blood Cells in Anemia. Increases *Vata*. Decreases *Pitta & Kapha*.

97

Table 7, continued

SUBSTANCE	TASTE	HEATING OR COOLING	POST-DIGESTIVE EFFECT	PROPERTIES & ACTION ON TRI-DOSHA
Herbs & Spices				
Anise Seed	Pungent	Heating	Pungent	Light. Promotes Digestion. Detoxifying Agent. Increases *Pitta*, Decreases *Vata & Kapha*.
Black Pepper	Pungent	Heating	Pungent	Light, Dry. Rough. Promotes Digestion. Increases *Pitta*, Stimulates *Vata*. Relieves *Kapha*.
Cardamom	Sweet & Pungent	Heating	Sweet	Promotes Digestion. Good for Heart. Improves Smell of Breath. May Stimulate *Pitta* if Taken in Excess. Relieves *Vata & Kapha*.
Celery Seed	Pungent	Heating	Pungent	Light. Helps Nausea. Increases *Pitta*. Decreases *Vata & Kapha*.
Cinnamon	Sweet, Bitter & Pungent	Heating	Sweet	Relieves Thirst. Stimulates Salivation. Relieves Dryness of Mouth. Stimulates *Kapha*. Decreases *Vata & Pitta*.
Clove	Pungent	Heating	Pungent	Promotes Digestion. Improves Taste & Flavor of Food. Increases *Pitta*. Decreases *Vata & Kapha*.
Coriander Seed	Pungent & Astringent	Cooling	Sweet	Oily, Dry, Light. Stops Burning Sensation of Urine. Helps Absorption. Increases *Vata & Kapha*. Relieves *Pitta*.
Cumin	Bitter, Pungent & Astringent	Heating	Pungent	Light, Oily, Smooth. Promotes Digestion. Relieves Diarrhea. Stimulates *Pitta*. Decreases *Vata & Kapha*.
Fenugreek (seed)	Bitter & Astringent	Heating	Pungent	Dry. Helpful for Fever & Arthritis. Increases *Vata & Pitta* if Taken in Excess. Decreases *Kapha*.

Name	Taste	Energy	Post-Digestive	Qualities / Actions
Garlic	Pungent	Heating	Pungent	Oily, Smooth, Heavy, Anti-Rheumatic. Good for Cough & Worms. Increases Pitta. Relieves *Vata* & *Kapha*.
Ginger (powder)	Pungent	Heating	Sweet	Light, Dry, Rough. Promotes Digestion. Detoxifying Agent. Increases Pitta if Taken in Excess. Relieves *Vata* & *Kapha*.
Mustard Seed	Pungent	Heating	Pungent	Oily, Light, Sharp. Relieves Muscular Pain. Increases Pitta. Decreases *Vata* & *Kapha*.
Saffron	Sweet & Astringent	Cooling	Sweet	Smooth, Relieves Hemorrhoids, Reduces Vomiting. Helps Stop Hemoptysis. Increases *Vata* & *Kapha*. Relieves *Pitta*.
Salt (general)	Salty	Heating	Sweet	Heavy, Rough. Promotes Digestion, Causes Retention of Water & Hypertension. Increases *Pitta* & *Kapha*. Relieves *Vata*.
Sesame (seed)	Sweet, Bitter & Astringent	Heating	Pungent	Heavy, Oily, Smooth, Strengthening. Increases *Pitta* & *Kapha*, Decreases *Vata*.
Turmeric	Bitter, Pungent & Astringent	Heating	Pungent	Helps in Diabetes, Promotes Digestion. Increases *Vata* & *Pitta* if Taken in Excess. Relieves *Kapha*.
Grains				
Barley	Sweet & Astringent	Cooling	Sweet	Light. Diuretic. Increases *Vata*. Decreases *Pitta* & *Kapha*.
Basmati Rice	Sweet	Cooling	Sweet	Light, Soft, Smooth, Nourishing. Decreases *Vata* & *Pitta*. OK for *Kapha* in small quantity.
Brown Rice	Sweet	Heating	Sweet	Heavy. Increases *Pitta* & *Kapha*, Decreases *Vata*.

Table 7, continued

SUBSTANCE	TASTE	HEATING OR COOLING	POST-DIGESTIVE EFFECT	PROPERTIES & ACTION ON TRI-DOSHA
Grains, *continued*				
Buckwheat	Sweet & Astringent	Heating	Sweet	Light & Dry. Increases *Vata & Pitta*. Decreases *Kapha*.
Corn (yellow)	Sweet	Heating	Sweet	Light, Dry. Increases *Vata & Pitta*. Reduces *Kapha*.
Millet	Sweet	Heating	Sweet	Light, Dry. Increases *Vata & Pitta*. Decreases *Kapha*.
Oats (dry)	Sweet	Heating	Sweet	Heavy. Dry Oats Increase *Vata & Pitta*. Reduces *Kapha*. Cooked Oats Increase *Kapha*. Reduce *Vata & Pitta*.
Rye	Sweet & Astringent	Heating	Sweet	Light, Dry. Increases *Vata & Pitta*. Reduces *Kapha*.
Wheat	Sweet	Cooling	Sweet	Heavy. Increases *Kapha*. Reduces *Vata & Pitta*.
White Rice (polished)	Sweet	Cooling	Sweet	Light, Soft, Smooth. Little nutrient value. OK for *Kapha* in small quantity. Reduces *Vata & Pitta*.
Nuts & Seeds				
Almond	Sweet	Heating	Sweet	Heavy, Oily. Increases *Pitta & Kapha*. Decreases *Vata*. Energizer. Aphrodisiac. Rejuvenator.
Cashew	Sweet	Heating	Sweet	Heavy, Oily. Increases *Pitta & Kapha*. Decreases *Vata*. Aphrodisiac.

	Rasa	Virya	Vipak	Properties & Action
Peanut	Sweet & Astringent	Heating	Sweet	Heavy, Oily. Increases *Pitta* & *Kapha*. OK for *Vata* in Moderation.
Pumpkin	Sweet, Bitter & Astringent	Heating	Pungent	Heavy, Dry. Kills Worms & Parasites. Increases *Pitta* & *Kapha*. Decreases *Vata*.
Sunflower	Sweet & Astringent	Heating	Sweet	Heavy, Oily. Slightly Increases *Pitta* & *Kapha*. Reduces *Vata*.
Walnut	Sweet & Astringent	Heating	Sweet	Heavy, Dry. Increases *Pitta* & *Kapha*. Decreases *Vata*.

Note: Foods have a long-term effect on the tri-dosha (see Table 5, pp. 82-84), while the properties and action of Rasa, Virya, Vipak have a brief effect on the tri-dosha.

CHAPTER X
Lifestyle and Routine

According to Ayurveda, routine plays a very important role in health. A natural life is a life regulated according to the individual constitution. It is best to have a daily regimen governing all daily actions such as the time one wakes up in the morning and the time one begins body purifications and meditation.

Early in the morning, preferably before sunrise, one should wake up, excrete waste products and clean the teeth and mouth. Next, one should look at the tongue, eyes, nose and throat and clean them. By examining the tongue, it is possible to detect pathological changes that may be occurring in the respective organs. After this examination, drinking a glass of warm water will help to clean the kidneys and large intestine. To clean the tongue, use a silver scraper. This process will serve to massage the tongue as well as the internal organs that correlate with the different areas of the tongue.

One should then massage the body with oil and take a bath. This will produce a sense of freshness and alertness. After the bath, put on comfortable clothes for exercise and meditation. Breathing exercises also are important in the daily regimen. After exercises, rest comfortably on the back with arms and legs outstretched and breathe from the lower abdomen.

Breakfast may follow exercise and meditation. Lunch should be eaten before noon, if possible, and dinner before sunset. It is best to go to bed before ten o'clock.

This regimen follows the flow of energy within the body and in the external environment. It is necessary at all times to remain aware of that flow in order to get the maximum benefit from your daily routine.

Other practices may be added to the routine depending on the individual constitution. For example, an oil massage is suggested in the evening for people of *vata* constitution.

Certain sleeping habits are advisable. Since the left side of a person contains female, or lunar, energy and the right side contains male, or solar, energy, the position in which one sleeps and breathes has a significant effect on the constitution and the balance of energies in the body.

If one always sleeps on the left side, it will suppress the lunar energy and aggravate the solar energy. The aggravation of solar energy may create *pitta* in the body. So, a person of *pitta* constitution should sleep on the right side. When one sleeps on the left side, lunar energy is suppressed and solar energy is opened. Sleeping in this position is recommended for *vata* and *kapha* types.

SUGGESTIONS FOR A CREATIVE, HEALTHY LIFE

Routine
- Awaken before sunrise.
- Evacuate bowels and bladder after awakening.
- Bathe every day to create a sense of bodily freshness.
- Twelve *pranayamas* in the morning or evening create freshness of mind and body.
- Do not take breakfast after 8:00 a.m.
- Wash hands before and after eating.
- Brush teeth after meals.
- Fifteen minutes after meals take a short walk.
- Eat in silence with awareness of food.
- Eat slowly.
- Each day massage the gums with the finger and sesame oil.
- Fast one day a week to help reduce toxins in the body.
- Sleep before 10:00 p.m.

Diet and Digestion
- One teaspoon of grated fresh ginger with a pinch of salt is a good appetizer.
- Drinking *lassi* (buttermilk) with a pinch of ginger or cumin powder helps digestion.
- A teaspoon of *ghee* with rice helps digestion.

- A glass of raw, warm milk with ginger taken at bedtime is nourishing to the body and calms the mind.
- Overeating is unhealthy.
- Drinking water immediately before or after taking food adversely affects digestion.
- Prolonged fasting is unhealthy.
- Consuming excess water may produce obesity.
- Excess intake of cold drinks reduces resistance and creates excess mucus.
- Store water in a copper vessel or put copper pennies in the water. This water is good for the liver and spleen.
- Taking a nap after lunch will increase *kapha* and body weight.

Physical Hygiene

- If possible, gaze at the rays of the sun at dawn for five minutes daily to improve eyesight.
- Gazing at a steady flame, morning and evening for ten minutes, improves eyesight.
- Do not repress the natural urges of the body, i.e., defecation, urination, coughing, sneezing, yawning, belching and passing gas.
- During a fever, do not eat and observe a ginger tea fast.
- Rubbing the soles of the feet with sesame oil before bedtime produces a calm, quiet sleep.
- Application of oil to the head calms the mind and induces sound sleep.
- Oil massage promotes circulation and relieves excess *vata*.
- Do not sleep on the belly.
- Reading in bed will injure the eyesight.
- Bad breath may indicate constipation, poor digestion, an unhygienic mouth and toxins in the colon.
- Body odor indicates toxins in the system.
- Lying on the back for fifteen minutes (*shavasan*) calms the mind and relaxes the body.
- Dry hair immediately after washing to prevent sinus problems.

- Blowing the nose forcibly may be injurious to the ears, eyes and nose.
- Continuous nose picking and scratching the anus may be a sign of worms in the body.
- Long fingernails may be unhygienic.
- Cracking the joints may be injurious to the body (causes deranged *vata*).
- Repeated masturbation may be injurious to the body (causes *vata* derangement).
- It is harmful to have sex during menstruation (causes deranged *vata*).
- After sex, milk heated with raw cashews and raw sugar promotes strength and maintains sexual energy.
- Oral and anal sex are unhygienic (cause *vata* derangement).
- Sex immediately after meals is injurious to the body.
- Avoid physical exertion such as yoga or running during menstruation.

Mental Hygiene
- Fear and nervousness dissipate energy and aggravate *vata*.
- Possessiveness, greed and attachment enhance *kapha*.
- Worry weakens the heart.
- Hate and anger create toxins in the body and aggravate *pitta*.
- Excessive talking dissipates energy and aggravates *vata*.

Sunrise - 10am Kapha
10am - 2pm Pitta
2pm - Sunset Vata
6pm - 10pm Kapha
10pm - 2am Pitta
2am - Sunrise Vata

CHAPTER XI

Time

T ime, like matter, is measurable. The substance of time moves and measurements exist to measure these movements: seconds, minutes, hours, days, weeks, months and years. There are also divisions of time within the day: morning, midday, afternoon, evening, midnight and dawn; and of the year into seasons.

Like time, the bodily humors are constantly in motion. There is a definite relationship between the movement of the *tridosha* and the movement or passage of time. The increase or decrease of these three humors in the body is related to the cycles of time. Morning, from sunrise till ten o'clock, is a time of *kapha*. Because of the predominance of *kapha* humor at this time, one feels energetic and fresh and also a little heavy. At mid-morning, *kapha* slowly merges into *pitta*. From ten in the morning till two in the afternoon is the time when *pitta* is secreted and hunger increases. One feels hungry, light and hot. The afternoon from two o'clock until the sun sets is the time of *vata* when one feels active, light and supple. Early in the evening from about six o'clock until ten is again *kapha* time, a period of cool air, inertia and little energy. Then from ten at night till two in the morning are the peak hours of *pitta* when food is digested. Early in the morning before sunrise is again *vata* time. Because *vata* creates movement, people awaken and excrete wastes.

Breakfast should be eaten early in the morning between about seven and eight o'clock. *Pitta* and *vata* people should eat breakfast; however, since eating at *kapha* time will increase *kapha* in the body, people of *kapha* constitution should not eat breakfast. The best time to eat lunch is at the beginning of *pitta* time between ten and eleven in the morning.

It is better to eat when the sun is up for the sun is the closest friend of man. Eating late at night will completely change the body chemistry; sleep will be disturbed and one will have unsettling dreams so that upon awakening one will not feel rested. If dinner is eaten at six o'clock, by nine the stomach will be empty and sleep will be sound. If the time of eating is changed so that meals are taken in keeping with the rhythm of the *tridosha*, a drastic change in one's living habits will occur.

Not only the time of day but also the seasons of the year are related to the movements of the *tridosha*. In the fall, September, October and November, the leaves fall, there is wind and the temperature begins to drop. At this time of year, *vata* predominates. Winter lasts from December to February. It is a time of clouds, snow and cold temperatures. This weather increases *kapha* and during this time colds, congestion, cough, bronchitis and pharyngitis are prevalent.

Spring, March through May, is the junction between winter and summer. *Kapha* is aggravated in early spring and *pitta* in the later part of spring. In early spring, the accumulated *kapha* of winter is liquified and slowly dries. The heat of the later spring increases the heat of *pitta* in the body, encouraging *pitta* disorders such as summer diarrhea, burning eyes, sunburn, hives, rash, dermatitis and burning feet.

It can be demonstrated, therefore, that changes in the time of day and season produce changes in the bodily humors, *vata*, *pitta* and *kapha*. Awareness of these changes helps one to keep in touch with the flow of energy in the external and internal environments.

SUN AND MOON

The concept of time encompasses not only the measurements of the clock and calendar, but also the phases of the moon and the flow of solar energy. All these changes relate to the bodily humors. The sun is related to human awareness or consciousness and the moon to the mind, which creates changes in emotions and mental faculties. The moon is the goddess of water which governs *kapha*. The moon's attributes are: cool, white, slow and dense. These are also attributes of *kapha*. During the full moon, *kapha* is aggravated in the body and the water element is stimulated in the external environment. At this time, the water in the ocean swells to create high

105

Chart 9
Tri-Dosha Mandala
Seasons & Times of Day

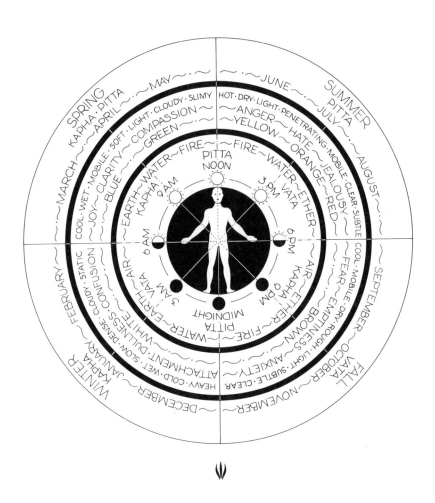

tides, which cause excess water in all life forms. People who have *kapha*-related asthma or *kapha*-related epilepsy will suffer more attacks during the full moon. Women have more menstrual cramps during the full moon.

At the time of the new moon, solar energy becomes intense. Because the energy of the sun is related to *pitta*, people who suffer from *pitta*-related epilepsy, for instance, will have more attacks during this time.

ASTROLOGY

Time also encompasses the movements of the planets. The planets are closely related to the bodily organs. Of all the concepts of time, astrological time is the most significant for the human nervous system because of the powerful influence of the planets on mind, body and consciousness.

Each planet is related to a specific bodily tissue. Mars, the red planet, is related to the blood and the liver. The liver is the seat of bile which is characterized by fire, *pitta*; and Mars influences the functioning of the liver and disorders that arise in that organ. This planet may also cause other *pitta* ailments such as increased toxins in the blood as well as hives and acne. Peptic ulcer and ulcerative colitis are aggravated by the effects of Mars.

Saturn is also a strong planet with profound effects. Its energy causes, for example, the wasting of muscle and emaciation. Venus is responsible for disorders of the semen, prostate gland, testicles and ovaries; while Mercury governs the reasoning capacity and its disorders. what about the other planets? List all.

AGES OF HUMAN LIFE

Time governs not only planetary movements but also the cycles of human life. The movement of time in the individual life is linked with a cycle of *vata-pitta-kapha*. Ayurveda teaches that there are three important milestones in the human lifetime: childhood, adulthood and old age. Childhood is the time of *kapha*, and children may suffer many *kapha* disorders such as lung congestion, cough, cold and mucus secretions. An infant's only food is mother's or cow's milk which may aggravate *kapha*. This time period of *kapha* lasts from birth until sixteen years.

Adulthood encompasses the years from sixteen to fifty. This period is the time of *pitta* when the individual is active and full of vitality. *Pitta* disorders are common at this time.

Old age is the time of *vata*. In old age, disorders will include *vata* ailments, such as tremors, emaciation, breathlessness, arthritis, loss of memory and wrinkles.

❧

CHAPTER XII
Longevity

From the time of physical birth until physical death, the body is engaged in a continuous struggle against the aging process. Because continuous breakdown of the bodily tissues and organs at the cellular level causes deterioration and degeneration, it is at the cellular level that rejuvenation must take place.

The *tridosha* play a very important role in the maintenance of cellular health and longevity. Each *dosha* plays a vital part in upholding the functioning of each of the billions of cells that constitute the human body. *Kapha* maintains longevity on the cellular level. *Pitta* governs digestion and nutrition. *Vata*, which is closely related to *pranic* life energy, governs all life functions.

On a deeper level, to combat aging it is necessary to balance the three subtle essences within the body: *prana, ojas* and *tejas*. The functioning of *prana, ojas* and *tejas* corresponds, at a subtler level of creation, to the functioning of *vata, kapha* and *pitta*, respectively. Proper diet, exercise and lifestyle can create a balance among these three subtle essences, ensuring long life.

Prana is the life energy that performs respiration, oxygenation and circulation. It also governs all the motor and sensory functions. The vital *pranic* force enkindles the central bodily fire (*agni*). Natural intelligence of the body is expressed spontaneously through *prana*. For example, if a child has a deficiency of iron or calcium, the body's natural intelligence, governed by *prana*, will lead the child to eat mud which is a source of these minerals.

The seat of *prana* is in the head and *prana* governs all higher cerebral activities. The functions of mind, memory, thought and emotions are all under the control of *prana*. The physiological functioning of the heart is also governed by *prana*, and from the heart *prana* enters the blood and thus controls oxygenation in all the *dhatus* and vital organs.

Prana governs the biological functions of the two other subtle

Ojas

essences, *ojas* and *tejas*. During pregnancy, the navel of the fetus is the main door through which *prana* enters the womb and the body of the fetus. This *prana* also regulates the circulation of *ojas* in the fetus. Thus, in all humans, even in the unborn, a disorder of *prana* may create an imbalance of *ojas* and *tejas* and vice-versa.

Ojas is the essence of the seven *dhatus* or bodily tissues. It is the vital energy that governs the hormonal balance. The super-fine element of *shukralartav* which is the essence of all *dhatus*, is located in the heart. Ojas is the vital energy that controls the life-functions with the help of *prana*. Ojas contains all of the five basic elements and all the vital substances of the bodily tissues. It is responsible for the auto-immune system and for mental intelligence.

Because *ojas* is related to kapha, aggravation of *kapha* displaces *ojas* and vice-versa. Displaced *ojas* creates the *kapha*-related disorders of diabetes, looseness of the bones and joints and numbness of the limbs. Decreased *ojas* will create *vata*-related reactions such as fear, general weakness, inability of the senses to perceive, loss of consciousness and death. Balanced *ojas* is necessary for biological strength and immunity.

Ghee helps to enhance *ojas*. Mother's milk promotes *ojas* in the body of the child so it is important that the child receive mother's milk in order to develop biological strength.

During the eighth month of pregnancy, *ojas* travels into the fetus from the body of the mother. Thus, if birth takes place prematurely before this transference of *ojas*, the baby will have difficulty surviving. This phenomenon demonstrates the importance of *ojas* in the maintenance of life functions. Just as *ojas* is necessary at the beginning of life, it is also necessary for longevity.

On the psychological level, *ojas* is responsible for compassion, love, peace and creativity. Through *pranayama*, spiritual discipline and *tantric* techniques, one can transform *ojas* into spiritual strength. This powerful spiritual energy creates an aura or halo around the crown *chakra*. A person with strong *ojas* is attractive, with lustrous eyes and a spontaneous and calming smile. Such an individual is full of spiritual energy and power. Spiritual practices and celibacy enhance these qualities in the individual. Those who indulge excessively in sex and masturbation dissipate *ojas* energy at the moment of orgasm. The result is weak *ojas* which directly affects the immune system. Such an individual becomes susceptible to psychosomatic ailments. See Recipe Section—Appendix C: *Almond Drink*.

Tejas is the essence of a very subtle fire that governs metabolism through the enzyme system. *Agni*, the central fire in the body, promotes digestion, absorption and assimilation of food. The further transformation of the ingredients of nutrition into the subtle tissues is governed by a subtle level of energy of *agni* — this is *tejas*. *Tejas* is necessary for the nourishing and transformation of each *dhatu*. Every *dhatu* has its own *tejas*, or *dhatu-agni*. This essence is responsible for the physiological functioning of the subtle tissues.

When *tejas* is aggravated, it burns away *ojas* reducing immunity and overstimulating *pranic* activity. Aggravated *prana* produces degenerative disorders in the *dhatus*. Lack of *tejas* results in overproduction of unhealthy tissue which creates growth of tumors and obstructs the flow of *pranic* energy.

Improper diet, bad living habits and overuse of drugs will cause an imbalance in *tejas*. Substances that are hot, sharp and penetrating directly enhance *tejas*.

Just as it is essential for health to ensure balance among the *tridosha*, the *dhatus* and the three *malas* or bodily wastes, it is also important for longevity that *prana*, *ojas* and *tejas* remain in balance. To create such balance, the rejuvenation process taught by Ayurveda is most effective.

Rejuvenation must take place on the physical, mental and spiritual levels. Before starting the physical rejuvenation program, the body must be cleansed. Just as dirty cloth will not take the right color when it is dyed, so the body will not profit from rejuvenation until it has first been cleaned from inside. A rejuvenating herb, taken orally, passes through the stomach, small intestine and large intestine before entering the bloodstream. All these physiological pathways must be purified in order for the herb to reach the deeper bodily tissues where the rejuvenation process begins.

Such bodily cleansings are accomplished by undertaking the five *pancha karma*: vomiting, purgatives, medicated enemas, nasal administration of herbs and purification of the blood. (For a detailed description of these treatments, see Chapter VII.) Vomiting cleanses the stomach which is the seat of *kapha*; purgation purifies the small intestine, the seat of *pitta*; medicated enemas cleanse the large intestine, the seat of *vata*; and nasal administration of herbs clarifies the mind and consciousness. To purify the blood, blood-letting is necessary; this treatment cleanses the blood so that the blood plasma may carry the rejuvenating nutrients of the herbs to the deep tissues.

Mental rejuvenation involves calming the mind. A quiet, meditative mind also helps to maintain longevity. Therefore, one must learn to "witness" all mental activities, thoughts and emotions, remaining detached from the experience. To promote mental peace, one Ayurvedic recommendation is isolation and avoidance of worldly affairs and society. However, this approach is not practical for most people. Hence, Ayurveda recommends a second method of mental rejuvenation, one in which the individual learns to be *in* the world but not *of* the world. With this approach, he observes his attachments to determine which of them creates stress. A life without attachment and stress is the happiest, healthiest and most peaceful one. Such a life creates natural longevity.

Celibacy and spiritual discipline also are useful for rejuvenation as are yogic practices. These disciplines lead to spiritual understanding and a healthfully altered way of living that promotes rejuvenation.

Modern medicine has developed the technology to sustain the life of the bodily functions, even after the communication of the body with the emotions and the spirit of the individual has ceased. Although Ayurveda supports the extension of life whenever possible, it also teaches that there may be *karmic* limitations to the life of an individual. Ayurveda respects both life and death and their intimate connection, and the science of life also suggests ways in which the individual can meet death peacefully. According to Ayurveda, death is a friend of man. The body dies; however, there is no death of the individual consciousness (soul): it is eternal.

To attain freedom, discipline is required. The Ayurvedic

foundations of discipline are a careful diet and a balanced way of living. Discipline of the body, mind and spirit is gained through pursuit of such traditional practices as *yoga*, *pranayama* and *tantra*. Such practices will bring man spiritual and physical freedom.

YOGA

According to Ayurveda, the practice of yoga, which is a spiritual science of life, is a very important, natural, preventive measure to ensure good health. Ayurveda and yoga are sister sciences. In India, it is traditional to study Ayurveda before taking up the practice of yoga, because Ayurveda is the science of the body and only when the body has become fit is the individual considered ready to study the spiritual science of yoga.

The yogic practices described by the father of yoga, Patanjali, are very useful in maintaining good health, happiness and longevity. Patanjali described the eight limbs of yoga and yogic practices. These are: the natural regulation of the nervous system; discipline; cleansing; postures; concentration; contemplation; the awakening of awareness; and the state of perfect equilibrium.

Yoga brings man to the natural state of tranquility which is equilibrium. Thus, yogic exercises have both preventive and curative value. Yogic practices help to bring natural order and balance to the neurohormones and the metabolism and improve the endocrine metabolism and thus provide fortification against stress. Yogic practices for the treatment of stress and stress-related disorders (such as hypertension, diabetes, asthma and obesity) are remarkably effective.

Yoga is the science of union with the Ultimate Being. Ayurveda is the science of living, of daily life. When yogis perform certain postures and follow certain disciplines, they open up and move energies that have accumulated and stagnated in the energy centers. When stagnant, these energies create various ailments. Yogis may temporarily suffer physical and psychological disorders because in the course of yogic cleansing of the mind, body and consciousness, disease-producing toxins are released. Employing Ayurvedic diagnoses and treatments, the yogis deal effectively with these disorders.

Ayurveda indicates which type of yoga is suitable for each person, according to his particular constitution. (The accompanying diagrams indicate which postures are good for each constitutional type as well as for specific disorders.) For example, a person of *pitta* constitution should not perform the headstand posture for more than one minute. If he does, the result will be mental disorientation. Similarly, a person of *vata* constitution should not perform the shoulder stand for a long time, because the shoulder stand exerts too much weight on the seventh cervical vertebra. This vertebra is sensitive and the delicate bone structure of *vata* may cause a shift in the spinal column. Repressed anger will shift the cervical vertebra to the right side and repressed fear will shift it to the left. The person of *kapha* constitution should not perform the hidden lotus posture for an extended time because this pose causes direct pressure on the adrenal glands.

BREATHING AND MEDITATION (Pranayama)

Breathing exercises, called *pranayama*, are a yogic healing technique that can bring about an extraordinary balance in the consciousness. In practicing *pranayama* one experiences Pure Being and learns the true meaning of peace and love. *Pranayama* has many healing benefits and also affects creativity. It can bring joy and bliss into life.

As with yoga, there are different types of *pranayama*. Ayurveda indicates which exercises are suitable for the different constitutional types. A person of *pitta* constitution should perform left nostril breathing. For this exercise, inhale through the left nostril and exhale through the right, using thumb and middle finger to close and open alternate nostrils. This exercise creates a cooling effect in the body by enhancing female energy.

A person of *kapha* constitution should do right nostril breathing, inhaling through the right nostril and exhaling through the left. This exercise creates a heating effect in the body by stimulating male energy.

A person of *vata* constitution should perform alternate nostril breathing. As *vata* is an active force, alternate nostril breathing brings

Chart 10
Yoga Postures for **V**ata, **P**itta, **K**apha Ailments

YOGA ASANAS FOR VATA

All postures should be performed while doing deep, quiet breathing.

1. **Vata Type of Asthma** - Backward Bend, Plough, Knee to Chest, Corpse

2. **Backache** - Knee to Chest, Plough, Half Wheel, Backward Bend

3. **Constipation** - Backward Bend, Yoga M*udra*, Knee to Chest, Shoulder Stand, Corpse. Belly should be drawn in while doing these postures.

4. **Depression** - Yoga M*udra*, Plough, Corpse, Palm Tree, Lotus

5. **Sciatica** - Knee to Chest, Backward Bend, Plough, Yoga M*udra*, Half Wheel

6. **Sexual Debility** - Backward Bend, Plough, Shoulder Stand, Elevated Lotus

7. **Varicose Veins** - Head Stand, Backward Bend, Corpse

8. **Wrinkles** - Yoga M*udra*, Backward Bend, Head Stand, Plough

9. **Rheumatoid Arthritis** - Half Wheel, Bow, Plough, Head Stand, Backward Bend

10. **Headache** - Plough, Yoga M*udra*, Head Stand

11. **Insomnia** - Corpse, Cobra, Backward Bend

12. **Menstrual Disorders** - Plough, Cobra, Half Wheel, Yoga M*udra*

YOGA ASANAS FOR PITTA

All postures should be performed while doing deep, quiet breathing

1. **Peptic Ulcer** - Hidden Lotus, *Sheetali* (inhale through coiled tongue through mouth)

2. **Hyperthyroidism** - Shoulder Stand, Ear Knee

3. **Malabsorption** - Knee to Chest, Fish, Locust

4. **Hypertension** - Shoulder Stand, Cobra, Half Bow, Quiet breathing

5. **Anger or Hate** - Half Bow, Shoulder Stand, Hidden Lotus, Corpse

6. **Migraine Headache** - *Sheetali*, Shoulder Stand, Fish

7. **Colitis** - Fish, Ear Knee, Boat, Bow

8. **Liver Disorder** - Fish, Shoulder Stand, Ear Knee, Hidden Lotus

9. **Hemorrhoids** - Fish, Shoulder Stand, Bow

10. **Stomatitis** (Inflammation of the Tongue) - *Sheetali*

YOGA ASANAS FOR KAPHA

All postures should be performed while doing, deep, quiet breathing.

1. **Bronchitis** - Head Stand, Plough, Forward Bend, Backward Bend, Half Wheel, Fish

2. **Emphysema** - Half Wheel, Shoulder Stand

3. **Sinus Congestion** - Fish, Boat, Plough, Bow, Breath of Fire (*Bhasrika*)

4. **Sinus Headache** - Lion, Head Knee, Fish

5. **Diabetes** - Boat, Fish, Half Wheel, Backward Bend, Forward Bend

6. **Chronic Gastro-Intestinal Disorders** - Fish, Locust, Cobra

7. **Sore Throat** - Lion, Shoulder Stand, Locust, Fish

8. **Asthma** - Half Wheel, Bow, Boat, Shoulder Stand, Palm Tree, Fish, Cobra

YOGA ASANAS

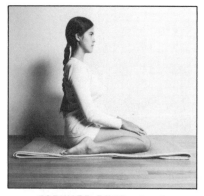
FORWARD BEND, step 1

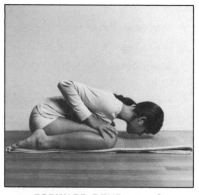
FORWARD BEND, step 2

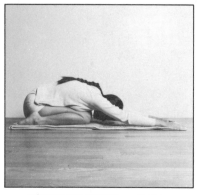
FORWARD BEND, variation

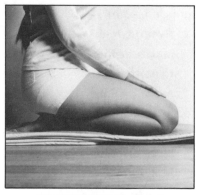
FORWARD BEND, detail

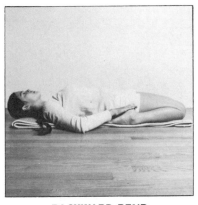

BACKWARD BEND

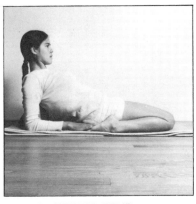

BACKWARD BEND, easy

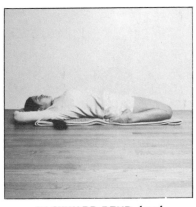

BACKWARD BEND, hard

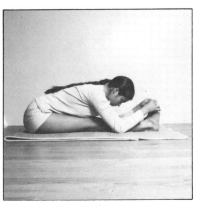

HEAD KNEE, correct

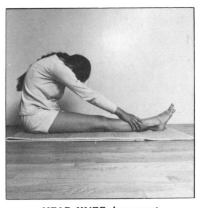

HEAD KNEE, incorrect

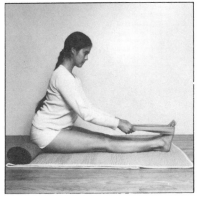

HEAD KNEE, assist

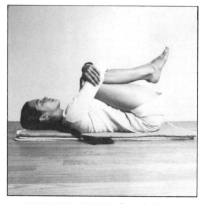

KNEE TO CHEST, head down

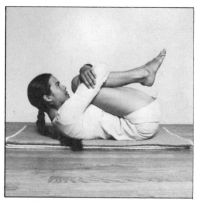

KNEE TO CHEST, head up

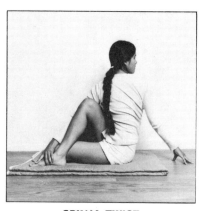

SPINAL TWIST

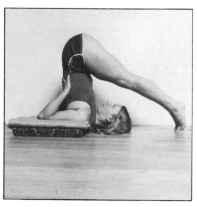

PLOUGH, correct

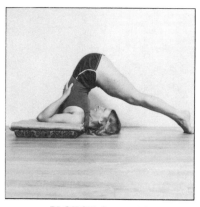

PLOUGH, incorrect

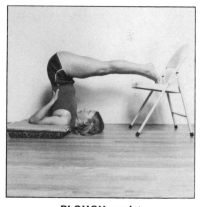

PLOUGH, assist

118

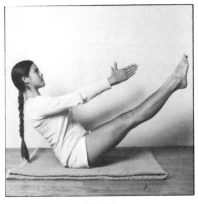

BOAT

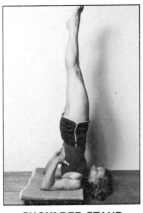

EAR KNEE

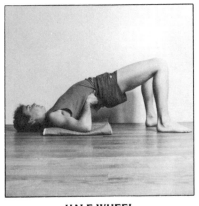

HALF WHEEL

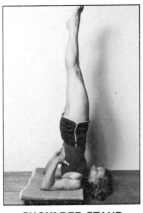

SHOULDER STAND

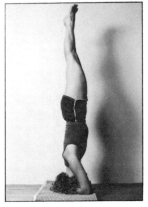

HEAD STAND

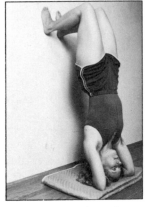

HEAD STAND, assist

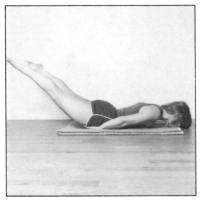

LOCUST

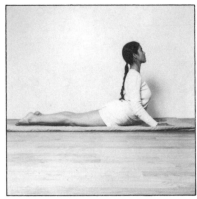

COBRA

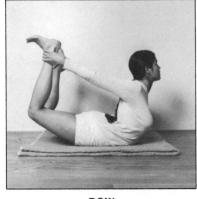

BOW

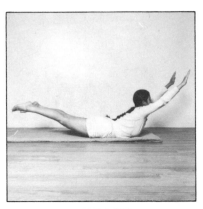

HALF BOW

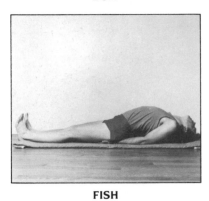

FISH

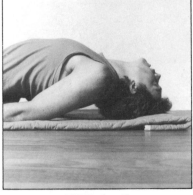

FISH, detail

120

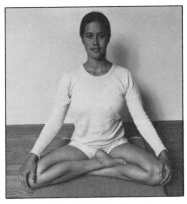

YOGA MUDRA, Step 1

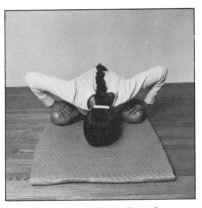

YOGA MUDRA, Step 2

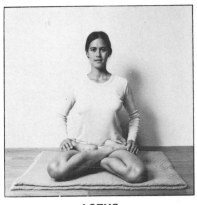

LOTUS

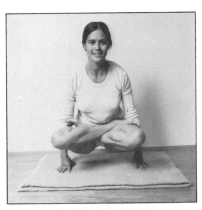

ELEVATED LOTUS

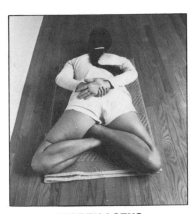

HIDDEN LOTUS

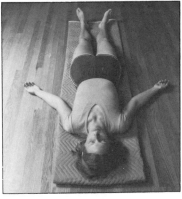

CORPSE

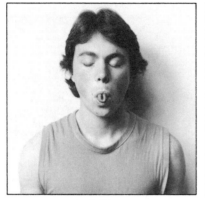

SHEETALI

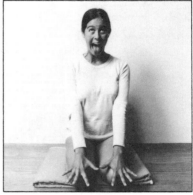

LION

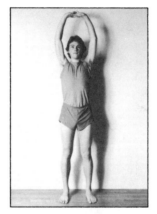

PALM TREE

balance.

One who is obese should perform the yogic breathing exercise called the 'breath of fire.' This exercise is done by sitting in a comfortable position, taking a deep breath and exhaling quickly and forcefully through the nose. Inhalation will happen naturally after each exhalation. This exercise aids in the metabolizing of fat. It should be performed for one full minute followed by one minute of rest and then another minute of breathing exercise for a total of five minutes. This exercise is the equivalent of running two miles.

Table 8
Asanas for Derangement of Vata, Pitta, Kapha

Dosha & Special Seat in the Body

VATA
Movement Producing Humour

Seat of Vata
Colon, Pelvic Cavity

VATA
Dry, Light, Cold,
Subtle, Rough, Moving,
Clear

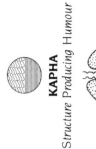

PITTA
Heat Producing Humour

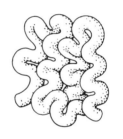

Seat of Pitta
Small Intestine

Qualities

PITTA
Oily, Sharp, Hot,
Light, Sour Smell,
Liquid, Fluid

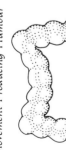

KAPHA
Structure Producing Humour

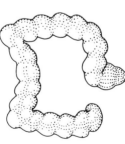

Seat of Kapha
Chest, Stomach

KAPHA
Cold, Oily, Heavy,
Slow, Steady, Smooth,
Dense

Asanas *that Balance Derangement of* Dosha

VATA

Asanas that place pressure on the pelvic and colon areas. Asanas done with slow, regular, silent breathing. Meditative asanas that put pressure on lower abdomen & make body well grounded. Balancing asanas that increase concentration making Prana smoother & finer.

LOTUS, BACKWARD BEND, HEAD KNEE, PLOUGH, LOCUST, CORPSE, COBRA, KNEE TO CHEST, HEAD STAND

PITTA

Asanas that affect the navel area, increase gastric heat efficiency & stimulate digestion. Asanas that stimulate liver, spleen & small intestines, & strengthen gastric fire (Agni).

HIDDEN LOTUS, EAR KNEE, BOW, FISH, SHOULDER STAND, HALF WHEEL, SHEETALI

KAPHA

Asanas that work on the chest, stomach & head areas bringing energy into the seat of Kapha. Strengthening asanas that increase flexibility & reduce fat and Kapha.

SPINAL TWIST, BOAT, LION, HEAD KNEE, PALM TREE, HALF WHEEL

124

(When an overweight person performs this breathing exercise, he will begin to sweat and become thirsty and then might desire a cold drink. Chilled drinks, however, should be avoided in this instance, because they will increase the build-up of fat in the body.)

Pranayama cleanses the lungs, heart and other organs and purifies the *nadis* which are *pranic* currents of energy in the body. Unless *pranayama* is performed carefully and systematically, it will create disorders in these delicate organs. *Pranayama* can cure disease when it is executed correctly; however, it will create disease if it is done improperly. The reader should not begin *pranayama* without the guidance of an individual who has experience in this yogic system of healing.

Mantra

Mantram (singular form) is a Sanskrit term denoting a word or group of words that carries certain phonetic vibrations and energy. Certain sacred Sanskrit words carry tremendous energy and chanting those sacred words in a prescribed manner releases this energy.

The chanting of a *mantram* should first be done aloud and sufficiently loudly so that one can listen to the sound. The vibration of the *mantram* penetrates deeper and deeper into the heart and finally one may remain silent, working internally with the supersonic sounds. This practice brings tremendous healing energy. The energy of a *mantram* helps one to achieve balance in the body, mind and consciousness. Just as food for the body should be chosen according to the constitution, so also with the *mantram* whose purpose and effective action is to nourish the individual soul.

Meditation

Meditation brings awareness, harmony and natural order to human life. It awakens the intelligence to make life happy, peaceful and creative. The awakening of this creative intelligence is the benediction of meditation. Let us share together a single, simple method of meditation.

Select free time, in the early morning if possible, and sit quietly.

Allow your eyes to survey the surrounding environment, your ears to receive its sounds. Relax your muscles. After spending some time observing this external world, close your eyes and bring your awareness from the outside to the inside.

Begin to notice the movements of your thoughts, desires and emotions. From the bank of consciousness observe the movements of the river of thoughts. Do not try to stop, change or place judgments on this experience. Through this internal observation, you are being cleansed of distractions; you are arriving at the beginning of a radical transformation. As unobstructed awareness increases, you will begin to enjoy increased relaxation and storehouses of energy will unlock within you: these are the benedictions of meditative practice.

Another form of meditation also brings great blessings. Sit quietly and observe your breathing. Breathing is the movement of *prana* and *prana* is life-force and life-energy which has two polarities: inspiration and expiration. Inspiration is cold and expiration warm. Together they create a natural biorhythm.

Through breathing, you will become aware of the vibration of cosmic sound. This cosmic sound, which is the soundless sound *aum*, has two manifestations, one male, the other female. The male manifestation is *hum* and the female energy is *so*. During inhalation, you will feel the vibration of the cosmic sound *so*. During exhalation, you will feel the sound *hum*.

In *so-hum* meditation, there is a union of individual consciousness with Cosmic Consciousness. Listen to the *so-hum, hum-so* sound through the breath. These vibrations are sound-energy which is one with the life-energy of the breath. Your breathing will become quiet and spontaneous and you will go beyond thought, beyond time and space, beyond cause and effect. Limitations will vanish; your consciousness will empty itself and in that emptying, consciousness will expand.

This merging of individual consciousness into the Cosmic Consciousness brings *samadhi*, the state of highest equilibrium. In that state, peace and joy will descend as a benediction. Your life will change and daily living will become a new and fresh exper-

Diagram 11
So-Hum Meditation

So (He)— Cosmic Consciousness
Hum (Me)— Individual Consciousness

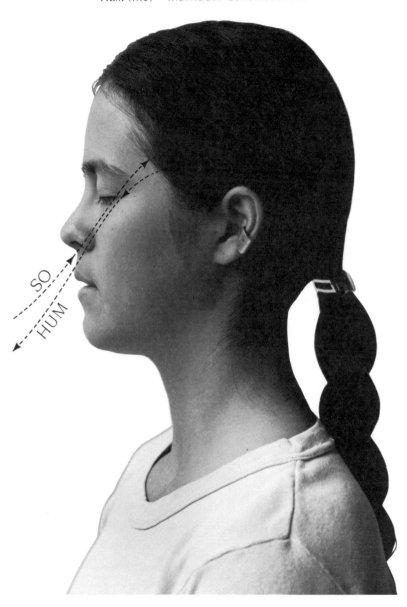

ience. Life will become meditation, for meditation is not separate from life but a part of life. Life is meditation and meditation is life. Creative intelligence will begin to operate in your body, mind and consciousness. All problems will dissolve in this new expanded awareness.

Meditation is necessary to bring harmony to one's daily living. Keep in mind, however, that the above-described results of meditation are the fruits only of committed and regular practice.

Massage

Massage is a therapy involved with movement of energy in the body. For the maintenance of health and to create balance among the three humors, *vata, pitta* and *kapha,* Ayurveda recommends massage with various oils. The massage process and type of oil depend upon the person's individual constitution.

For an aggravated *vata* condition, Ayurveda suggests massage with sesame oil to calm and balance the body. Stroking against the grain of body hairs facilitates penetration of the oil into the hair follicles. This technique is indicated because *vata* people have dry skin and closed follicles. Massage for a person of *pitta* constitution should be done with sunflower or sandalwood oil because these have cooling properties. For *kapha* constitution, one can use corn or calamus root oil or the massage can be given without oil.

Certain techniques apply to specific disorders. For example, for stagnation of blood and poor circulation, massage toward the heart. For muscle spasms, tightness and soreness, massage in the direction of muscle fibers. Massage should be done in the morning during *kapha* time for *kapha* disorders, in the evening for *vata* disorders and in the afternoon for *pitta* disorders. For *kapha* people, deep massage is beneficial. A gentle massage is good for *vata* and *pitta* individuals.

CHAPTER XIII
Medicinals

The pharmacology of Ayurveda is a vast science including
thousands of medicines, many of them herbal prepara-
tions. In addition to these herbal cures, remedies less familiar in the West such as the use of the healing properties of gems,
metals and colors are recommended. The classic Ayurvedic texts
state that all substances found in nature have medicinal value when
used in the proper manner. The purpose of these remedies is not to
suppress the effects of illness as is often the case in Western
medicine, but rather to bring the out-of-balance factors in the body
into harmony once more, thereby eliminating the cause of disease.
The purpose and action of Ayurvedic remedies are to eradicate the
disease itself, not just the symptoms of illness.

Ayurveda is a very practical science and the advice that
follows, suggesting simple treatments for minor ailments and util-
izing herbs commonly found in the kitchen, is straightforward and
effective. At least eighty percent of all diseases are self-limiting:
that is, if nothing is done to alter the disease process, the body's
own mechanisms will eventually restore the nervous system to a
state of health. The information in this chapter specifically indicates
methods to support the body in its natural process of balancing the
internal and external environments, thus promoting healing.

Of course, if the ailment or disease does not subside, after application of these methods, a physician should be consulted. At times
symptoms that appear minor may have serious repercussions.

The Kitchen Pharmacy

The kitchen can become your domestic clinic. You can use
your kitchen and its resources to create herbal cures that will heal
your family and yourself. The following are commonly-available
natural substances that may be employed in the home.

Alfalfa. This herb has an astringent and slightly bitter taste. It has anti-*vata* and anti-*kapha* properties and is also anti-inflammatory. It is very effective in cleansing toxins from the large intestine. Alfalfa is a natural pain reliever and may be used to treat such diseases as sciatica. Alfalfa tea can be taken at bedtime for arthritis, rheumatism, colitis, ulcers and anemia.

Aloe vera. This common herb is universally available. It is a general tonic for the liver, the organ that aids digestion and neutralizes toxins. Its effects are anti-*vata*, anti-*pitta* and anti-*kapha*, so it will not aggravate any humor in the body. Aloe vera helps to balance *vata, pitta* and *kapha* in the body.

The fresh gel of aloe vera is useful for women who have muscle spasms during menstruation. For this discomfort, one or two teaspoons of the gel should be taken with a pinch of black pepper. Two teaspoons three times a day may be used as a general tonic. Aloe vera is a blood purifier and in this way benefits the liver, gallbladder and stomach. It is also helpful in cases of ulcers and colitis and it relieves inflammation. One can also apply aloe vera gel directly to the outer eyelid for conjunctivitis.

Aloe vera may be used for vaginitis or cervicitis. Prepare a douche of two tablespoons of the gel in one quart of warm water and add two pinches of turmeric to the solution. This douche should be used every other day for four days. It has a highly effective local action.

Aloe vera has a cooling property; however, it does not aggravate *kapha* because its action causes expectoration. It can relieve colds, coughs and congestion and is also a mild laxative.

Aloe vera also may be used externally for burns, cuts and traumatic wounds. Apply it with turmeric which helps the healing process. Local application is also useful for vaginal herpes. For the symptomatic relief of herpes, mix two tablespoons of gel with two pinches of turmeric. Apply locally every night at bedtime for one week.

Asafoetida. This aromatic substance, which is a gum extract from a tree, is a stimulant. It also relieves spasms. It is a good expectorant and natural laxative.

A pinch of asafoetida cooked with lentils helps digestion. It enkindles *agni*, removes toxins and relieves pain. It also relieves gas in the large intestine.

If there is pain in the ear, a little asafoetida wrapped in a piece of cotton may be placed in the ear. Its odor will relieve the pain.

Baking soda. When cooked with garbanzo or black beans, baking soda makes them lighter and facilitates the cooking process. It is also an antacid. A pinchful with one cup of warm water and the juice of one-half lemon relieves acidity, gas and indigestion. Half a cup of baking soda in the bath helps circulation and makes the skin soft. Baking soda relieves skin infections, hives and rash and maintains the health and hygiene of the skin.

Calamus root. This herb is hot and penetrating and is used as an expectorant. It is also an emetic.

Calamus root has many medicinal properties. As a powder, it may be taken into the nose like snuff to relieve sinus congestion, common cold or sinus headache. It may create sneezing which will cleanse the respiratory tract.

According to Ayurveda, calamus is anticonvulsive. It is used for epileptic seizures. It acts on the higher cerebral functions and brain tissue to help expand and bring clarity to the consciousness. Calamus root is the best antidote for the ill effects of marijuana. Marijuana is toxic to the liver and the brain cells; however, if one smokes a pinch of calamus root powder with the marijuana, this herb will completely neutralize the toxic side effects of the drug. In fact, the side effects of all psychedelics can be neutralized by calamus root.

To promote the intelligence of a growing child, heat a golden wire and insert it into the center of a calamus root stick along the axis. Then rub this preparation on a rough stone and mix it with mother's milk. Give the child one-half to one teaspoonful of this remedy. It will also protect the child from *kapha* disorders.

Calamus root is also used to improve the memory. In the morning and evening, take a pinch of the powdered root with one-fourth to one-half teaspoonful of honey.

If one drinks two to three glasses of calamus root tea, it will cause vomiting. This action is therapeutic for chronic cough and asthma. Calamus root is also a broncho-dilator and acts as a chest decongestant.

The medicated oil of calamus root may be used for nasal administration and also externally for massages to relieve *vata* and *kapha* disorders. Massaging with this oil will relax tense and sore muscles and create a feeling of freshness. Calamus root helps the circulation and provides nutrition for the muscle tissue.

Cardamom. Cardamom is aromatic, stimulating and refreshing. It also enkindles digestive fire. It refreshes the mind and is a heart stimulant.

Cardamom is slightly astringent, sweet and a little pungent. It should be used only in small quantities, sprinkled in tea or on vegetables.

Cardamom strengthens the heart and lungs. It also relieves gas. It is a pain reliever and it sharpens the mind, opens the breathing and freshens the breath.

Castor oil. This substance is a laxative that is safe enough to use even in treating small babies. (To treat an infant, the mother should dip her little finger into the oil and let the baby suck on it.) For chronic constipation, one tablespoon of castor oil should be taken with a cup of ginger tea. This tonic will neutralize toxins and relieve gas and constipation.

Castor oil is also an antirheumatic herb because it is a natural pain reliever and laxative.

The tea of the castor root is used in treating many *vata* disorders, such as arthritis, sciatica, chronic backache and muscle spasms. The tea is also a decongestant, anti-arthritic and anti-inflammatory substance. It is also effective in the treatment of gout.

Cayenne pepper. This spice is pungent and hot. It is a domestic herb which is used in cooking. It enkindles digestive fire and is a good appetizer. It enhances circulation and causes sweating. Cayenne helps to evacuate the bowel and destroys worms and parasites. It is good for colds, cough and congestion.

Cayenne has a cleansing action upon the large intestine and sweat glands. It may be used internally by placing the cayenne in 00 capsulés. Two capsules two to three times a day help to break down blood clots. It is good for *vata* and *kapha* disorders but not for those of *pitta*. Cayenne helps to reduce the heaviness of food and makes it light, palatable and easily absorbable. It should be used with meat, lentils and cheese.

Cinnamon. This herb is aromatic and is a stimulant with anti-septic and refreshing properties. The taste is slightly pungent and astringent. The action on the body is hot.

Cinnamon is a good detoxifying herb. It creates freshness and strengthens and energizes the tissues. Cinnamon also acts as a pain reliever. It relieves *vata* and *kapha* disorders and can also be used in *pitta* ailments if taken in small quantities. However, if it is taken in excess, it will disturb *pitta*.

Cinnamon enkindles *agni*, promotes digestion and has a natural cleansing action. It also stimulates sweating. It is good for the relief of colds, congestion and cough. Cinnamon, cardamom, ginger and clove are used together as a tea to relieve cough and congestion and to promote digestion. It should be taken in small quantities, one pinch at a time.

Cloves. This is another aromatic herbal substance. It is hot, pungent, oily and sharp. Therefore, it aggravates *pitta*. Cloves will help to control *vata* and *kapha*.

Cloves may be used in powder form with vegetables and fruits. Powdered cloves also may be taken as a tea. Adding a pinch of powdered cloves to ginger tea will relieve *vata* and *kapha*.

Cloves are a natural pain reliever. Oil of cloves is used to relieve toothache. For this treatment, a small piece of cotton is dipped into the oil and inserted into the cavity of the tooth.

Cloves will alleviate coughs, congestion, colds and sinus problems. A few drops of clove oil may be added to boiling water and the fumes may then be inhaled as a decongestant. This will relieve nasal obstruction and congestion.

Chewing a piece of clove with rock candy helps to alleviate a dry cough. (Rock candy is recommended so that *pitta* will not be aggravated since clove is hot and will create a burning sensation on the tongue.)

Coriander. There are two forms of coriander. One is the fresh greens of the plant; these are called *cilantro*. The other is the dry seed which is coriander. This is an aromatic and stimulating substance that aids digestion. It also has a cooling property. Coriander is a natural diuretic and it may be taken when one feels a burning sensation while passing urine. For this treatment, prepare a tea from the seeds and pour hot water over a strainer in the water to make an infusion. This tea makes the urine more alkaline. It is also useful for gas, indigestion, nausea and vomiting.

Fresh coriander juice has anti-*pitta* properties and is used for rash, hives and dermatitis. It may be applied as a pulp to the skin to relieve a burning sensation. It also helps to purify the blood.

Cumin. This herb is aromatic and slightly bitter and pungent. It helps digestion and improves the taste of food. It also aids the secretion of digestive juices.

Roasted cumin powder is effectively used in intestinal disorders such as diarrhea or dysentery. For such ailments, a pinch of cumin powder is taken with freshly-prepared buttermilk (see recipe section — Appendix C).

Cumin also relieves pain and cramps in the abdomen. It is very effective for *pitta* and *kapha* disorders.

Flax seeds. The actions of flax seeds are: laxative, expectorant and decongestant. Flax tea is recommended for these disorders. If one cup of this tea is taken at night, the bowels will move easily in the morning. It will also aid the drainage of mucus through the feces.

This simple domestic herb also alleviates the problems of constipation, distention and discomfort in the abdominal region. Flax seeds are energizing and also help in relieving asthma and chronic cough.

Garlic. This herb contains oil; it is aromatic, hot, bitter and pungent. Garlic relieves aggravated *vata* and alleviates gas. It is good for digestion and absorption and is also a good rejuvenating herb.

Many spiritual people say that garlic is "*rajas*" (inhibits spiritual growth), and should not be taken by spiritual practitioners. Garlic does stimulate sexual energy and is, therefore, not recommended for those who practice celibacy.

Apart from its spiritual contraindications, garlic is very effective for *vata* disorders. Since it has a warming effect, it is helpful during the rainy season and the winter. It also relieves pain in the joints. However, garlic is not good for people of *pitta* constitution because of its hot and pungent attributes.

This herb is anti-rheumatic and may be used for a dry cough or congestion. It is very effective for sinus headaches and pain or tingling in the ear. In treating ear problems, three to four drops of garlic oil are placed in the ear, or the ear is filled with this oil at night and sealed with cotton. By morning the pain will have disappeared.

Garlic will also relieve toothache. Sensitive teeth or receding gums may be massaged with garlic oil.

Fresh garlic may be used for cooking. It makes the food more palatable and easier to absorb and it enkindles *agni*. Fresh garlic is anti-*vata* and anti-*kapha*.

Ghee. Ghee is a product made from unsalted butter (see recipe section — Appendix C). It is an excellent appetizer, enkindling *agni*, and it enhances the flavor of foods. It also helps digestion because it stimulates the secretion of digestive juices. *Ghee* also helps to enhance intelligence, understanding, memory and *ojas*. It relieves constipation if taken with warm milk. When used with various herbs, *ghee* carries their medicinal properties to the tissues. Combined with licorice, calamus root or gotu kola, it is used extensively as an Ayurvedic medicinal (see recipe section — Appendix C).

Ghee relieves chronic fever, anemia and blood disorders and is useful for detoxification. It does not increase cholesterol as do many other oils and it has anti-*vata*, anti-*pitta* and anti-*kapha* properties. Thus it aids in the balancing of the *tridosha*. *Ghee* promotes the healing of wounds and alleviates peptic ulcer and colitis. It is good generally for the eyes, nose and skin.

Ginger This herb is used fresh and dried. Both forms of the herb are aromatic and pungent. Ginger is a stimulant and a carminative. Fresh ginger contains more water and is milder; the powdered form is stronger and has more penetrating action.

Fresh ginger tea is good for *vata* and *pitta* people. Dry ginger, being highly concentrated and strong, is good for *kapha* people. Ginger causes sweating, enkindles *agni*, neutralizes toxins and helps digestion, absorption and assimilation of food. Ginger alleviates inflammation of the throat, the common cold, congestion and sinus problems. A tea of ginger powder mixed with hot water may be taken with honey.

Grated fresh ginger with a little garlic can be eaten to counteract low *agni*. This concoction will enkindle *agni* so that the appetite returns. A pinchful of salt added to one-half teaspoonful of grated fresh ginger also acts as an excellent appetizer.

Ginger is the best domestic remedy for *kapha* problems such as cough, runny nose, congestion and throat congestion.

To alleviate headaches, prepare a paste of one-half teaspoonful of ginger powder mixed with water and heated and apply it to the forehead. This paste will create a slight burning sensation but will not burn the skin and it will relieve the headache.

Ginger may also be used as a spice in cooking. It is especially helpful in cold weather. Ginger makes food lighter and easier to digest. It will aid in cleansing the intestines and will promote healthy bowel movements.

Ginger also may be applied externally to painful joints and muscles. It helps the circulation and relieves pain by causing stagnant energy to be released.

For body aches, a ginger bath is recommended. Grated ginger is placed in a piece of cloth and tied to the hot water tap so that the hot water flows through the ginger. This ginger-water relieves pain and has a refreshing and relaxing effect.

Gotu kola. The leaf of the gotu kola herb looks like the two hemispheres of the brain. Gotu kola acts upon the brain tissue. It is a very effective aid for developing memory and intelligence. It stimulates the brain tissues, thereby expanding understanding and comprehension.

Gotu kola relieves stress and calms the mind. In Sanskrit, it is called *brahmi* (*Brahma* means Cosmic Consciousness). This herb will help the flow of energy in the brain between the right and left hemispheres.

Gotu kola also is a decongestant and is used to alleviate sinus problems. To cleanse mucus, use the powder form: take one-fourth teaspoonful with honey, morning and evening.

Gotu kola's essential action is upon the mind and higher consciousness. One also may take it in the form of a tea, one cup at bedtime, to promote sound sleep and peaceful, alert awakening.

Honey. This substance creates heat in the body; therefore it acts to reduce *vata* and *kapha.* Its taste is sweet and astringent. Honey is good for healing internal and external ulcers. Like ghee, honey carries the medicinal properties of herbs to the bodily tissues and is, therefore, used as a medium for many substances. Honey is an excellent blood purifier and is also good for the eyes and teeth. It alleviates cold, cough and congestion. When used to dress an external wound, it will help the healing process.

Honey and water together energize the body and help to flush the kidneys. If taken in moderation, it reduces fat. Honey should not be cooked because cooking alters its attributes and makes it incompatible with the body. Heated honey can clog the digestive tract and create toxins.

Licorice. This substance is sweet and slightly astringent. It is a natural expectorant. Licorice cleanses the mouth, promotes salivation and increases secretions in the gastrointestinal tract. Chewing on a licorice stick will clean the mouth and cleanse the teeth, arresting tooth decay. Licorice also has a germicidal action.

It also is used to alleviate coughs, colds and congestion. For these purposes it is taken as a tea to aid in expectoration.

Licorice is also an emetic. Two to three glasses of strong licorice tea will cause nausea and vomiting which helps to remove excess mucus accumulated in the stomach and also the excess mucus which creates congestion in the chest.

Licorice is a very effective antidote for peptic ulcers and gastritis. For treating these ailments, use one teaspoonful or less of licorice powder in preparing one cup of tea.

Licorice may be made into a medicated oil or medicated with *ghee* for internal use. This medicinal is used for diabetes, bronchitis, cold and repeated attacks of asthma. (See licorice *ghee* preparation in recipe section — Appendix C.)

Licorice *ghee* may be used externally on wounds. Septic or non-healing wounds will be healed by the application of licorice *ghee*. If one takes licorice *ghee* regularly (one-half teaspoon every day), it helps to relieve the inflammation of peptic ulcers.

Licorice also is a very effective antidote for inflammation of the gallbladder. Taken after meals, licorice tea aids digestion and relieves constipation.

Mustard. Mustard is very pungent, hot, sharp, penetrating and oily. The seed is used as a domestic spice. It enkindles *agni* and neutralizes toxins. However, mustard must be used with care because it aggravates *pitta*.

Mustard acts as an analgesic and it reduces muscular pain. It is a carminative and also relieves congestion.

Mustard powder mixed with water may be used as a poultice. It should not be applied directly to the skin or blistering may occur. The paste should be applied to a cloth and the cloth placed next to the skin for relief of painful joints or pain in the chest.

Mustard also may be used as a fomentation to relieve muscle spasms. Tie the mustard seeds in a small cloth and place the cloth in hot water. Then immerse the hands and feet in the water for relief of joint pain or muscle soreness. Mustard seeds mixed with water relax the muscles.

Mustard may be used in cooking and frying. Heat sesame oil in a pan; when the oil is hot, fry approximately two pinches of mustard seed with onion, garlic and vegetables. The vegetables then become very light and easy to digest. Mustard may be used for indigestion, distention of the abdomen and discomfort caused by improper digestion.

Nutmeg. This herb is aromatic and stimulating. It is used to improve the taste of teas and milk. When taken with milk, it serves as a tonic for the heart and brain. It is also used to alleviate sexual debility. Nutmeg also is effective in treating lack of control over urination, general weakness, diarrhea, gas and dull aching pain in the abdomen as well as loss of appetite and liver and spleen disorders.

Nutmeg is a relaxant and it induces natural sleep; thus it is helpful for insomnia. It should be taken sparingly and only by adults because of its strong action — one pinchful at a time.

It is very good for *vata* or *kapha* people. For people of *pitta* constitution, nutmeg may be used in smaller doses.

Onion. The onion is a strong irritant and is pungent and aromatic. Its action is hot when taken internally. The fumes contain ammonia, are an irritant to the eyes and cause the nose and eyes to run. Onions stimulate the senses so if one feels faint or dizzy, an onion broken into pieces and inhaled will bring relief. Onions help the digestion and stimulate sexual energy. They are *rajas* food and are not recommended to those who practice celibacy as a spiritual discipline.

Cooked onions are sweet and less pungent. If they are applied as a poultice to a skin boil, the boil will burst. High fever and resultant convulsions may be relieved by applying a grated raw onion wrapped in a piece of cloth to either the forehead or abdomen.

Onions will relieve acute epileptic seizures if applied as a nasal inhalent or as eye drops. They also help to reduce cholesterol and are a good heart tonic: the action of onions helps reduce the heart rate. One-half cup of fresh onion juice with two teaspoons of honey taken internally, relieves asthma, cough, spasms, nausea and vomiting. It also will destroy intestinal worms. A grated onion with one-half teaspoonful of turmeric and one-half teaspoonful of curry powder will relieve pain in the joints when applied as a paste to the affected area.

Pepper (black). This spice is pungent and hot and is a stimulant that helps to enkindle *agni.* It increases the secretion of digestive juices and improves the taste of food. It is used to alleviate con-stipation, dry hemorrhoids, gas and loss of appetite. This herb also may be taken with a pinch of honey to combat worms in the large intestine. Ground, whole peppercorns should be used only.

Black pepper helps to relieve swelling. As an antidote to hives, a pinch of black pepper powder with *ghee* is applied externally. Black pepper is hot and pungent, but mixed with *ghee* it relieves *pitta* disorders such as dermatitis and hives.

Salt. Many people use sea salt simply to improve the taste of food; however, it also has medicinal properties. Salt contains water and is a by-product of the sea. It aggravates *pitta* and *kapha* because it contains water and fire. Only small amounts should be used in cooking.

Salt relieves gas and distention of the abdomen. It cleanses the mouth, stimulates secretions in the digestive canal and aids digestion.

Salt may be used to relieve external swellings. The salt should be heated in a pan and placed in a cloth bag. It may then be applied externally. Salt also is a natural pain reliever and may be used exter-nally as a local application for pain. It helps to increase drainage: put a few drops of a concentrated salt solution into the nose to cleanse *kapha* and relieve nasal blockage.

Turmeric. This herb is aromatic and a stimulant and has many helpful functions. It is bitter, slightly pungent and a good blood purifier, and works as a tonic to aid digestion and relieve congestion. It has a soothing action on respiratory ailments such as cough and asthma. It also is antiarthritic and acts as a natural anti-bacterial.

Turmeric may be added to high-protein food to assist digestion and prevent the formation of gas. It is effectively used to maintain the flora of the large intestine.

To relieve inflammation of the tonsils and congestion in the throat, turmeric also may be used as a gargle: for this purpose, mix two pinches of turmeric and two pinches of salt in a glass of hot water.

Turmeric also has anti-inflammatory properties. For an abrasion, bruise or traumatic swelling, turmeric paste may be applied locally. To one-half teaspoonful of turmeric add a pinch of salt and apply to the affected area. Pain, swelling and inflammation will be quickly relieved.

For the treatment of diabetes, turmeric is also useful. Take four to five 00 capsules after each meal to help return the blood sugar level to normal.

Yellow dock. This herb is a famous native of America. It has anti-*pitta* properties. It is a laxative, purifies the blood and is also anti-inflammatory. Hence, it may be used for arthritis symptoms and the alleviation of pain, tenderness and redness. It also is effective, used in tea form, for dermatitis, bleeding hemorrhoids and inflammatory eruptions on the neck and back and in the armpits.

Because of its antitoxic property, yellow dock purifies the blood and calms out-of-balance *pitta*. The root of this herb is useful for external application to ulcers, skin infections and poorly healed abrasions.

Metals *

In addition to the use of herbs as medicinals, Ayurveda utilizes

*Caution: The following metals have potentially toxic effects when used to excess. They should only be used under the supervision of a qualified Ayurvedic physician.

the healing properties of metals, gems and stones. Ayurvedic teachings hold that everything in existence is endowed with the energy of Universal Consciousness. All forms of matter are simply the outer manifestations of this energy. *Prana*, the vital force of life, flows from this universal energy which is the essence of all matter. Thus, metals, stones and gems are the outer manifestations of certain forms of energy and these materials contain *pranic* energy reservoirs that may be drawn upon for healing purposes. The ancient *rishis* of India discovered these healing energy-effects through meditation.

Adverse influences upon the normal functions of the body, mind and consciousness may be counteracted through the use of gems and metals. When they are applied to the skin, they induce an electromagnetic influence that acts upon the physical cells and deeper tissues. For example, by wearing an armlet of silver and lead, one may avoid impending liver trouble.

Physical health depends on cosmic influences as well as the spiritual and mental state of the individual. As a house is protected from lightning by a copper rod, so the body may be protected from electrical and magnetic radiation in the atmosphere through the use of gems and metals. Pure metals emit an astral light that provides a powerful counteraction to the negative pull of the planets.

All metals contain tremendous healing energy. The heavy metals, such as mercury, gold; silver, copper,iron, lead and tin are used in healing. However, even pure metals may contain certain impurities that are toxic to the vital organs, such as the kidney, liver, spleen and heart. Therefore, the Ayurvedic teachings prescribe specific methods for their purification. The metal is heated and treated with oil, cow's urine, milk, ghee, buttermilk or the sour gruel of grains. These ancient methods achieve subtler purification than mere chemical treatments and permit the human tissues to receive the metals' influences without any toxic effects. The beneficial effects of several metals will now be described.

Copper: alleviates excess *kapha* and fat. It is a good tonic for the liver, spleen and lymphatic system. It is especially useful for the person who tends to put on weight, retains water or has a lymphatic obstruction. It is also helpful in curing anemia.

To treat obesity and liver and spleen disorders, wash ten pennies in lime water, place them in one quart of water and boil until half the water remains. Two teaspoonsful of this copper-water should be taken three times a day for one month. It is also helpful to wear a copper bracelet on the wrist.

Gold: is an effective nervine tonic. It improves memory and intelligence, strengthens the heart muscle and increases stamina. Gold is good for hysteria, epilepsy, heart attacks, weak lungs and spleen.

Purified gold is turned into ash by burning it in a fire. The energy of gold also may be harnessed through the use of gold-medicated water. To prepare such water, place a golden ornament (without any stone) into two glasses of water and boil until half the water evaporates. The electronic energy of the gold will enter the water during this process. One teaspoonful of this water may be taken two or three times a day. Gold water will energize the heart causing a feeble pulse to become strong. It also will improve memory, intelligence and comprehension and stimulate awakening awareness.

Gold has hot properties and therefore should be used cautiously if one has a *pitta* constitution. Some people will not tolerate gold and may break out in a rash if gold is applied.

Iron: is beneficial for bone marrow, bone tissue, red blood cells, liver and spleen. It increases the production of red blood cells and therefore the ash is used to treat anemia. It is effectively used as an antidote for enlargement of the liver or spleen. Iron strengthens muscle and nerve tissues and has rejuvenating properties.

Lead: is a very effective medicinal for skin diseases. It is used also to treat leukorrhea, vaginal discharge, swelling, gonorrhea and syphilis.

Mercury: is a very heavy and potent metal. It helps to enkindle the enzyme system and transforms and regenerates the tissues. Mercury is considered the semen of the god *Shiva* in Indian mythology. It stimulates intelligence and awakens awareness. It should never be used alone, but always in conjunction with sulphur. The potency of certain herbs is increased many thousandfold when used in conjunction with mercury and sulphur. These two metals carry the actions of the herbs to the subtle channels and tissues of the body.

Silver: is another very important healing metal. Silver has cooling properties so it is beneficial for treating excess *pitta*. Silver promotes strength and stamina. It also may be used for the treatment of *vata* ailments; however, silver should be used with caution in treating *kapha* people. Silver is helpful for emaciation, chronic fever, weakness after fever, heartburn, inflammatory conditions of the intestines, hyperactivity of the gallbladder and profuse menstrual bleeding. Silver ash is very useful in alleviating inflammatory heart diseases and liver and spleen disorders.

Silver water is prepared by the same method as gold water. Drink warm milk heated in a silver container to improve strength and stamina.

Tin: is a natural rejuvenating element. The purified ash of tin is used in treating diabetes, gonorrhea, syphilis, asthma, respiratory infection, anemia, skin diseases, lung diseases and lymphatic obstructions.

GEMS, STONES AND COLOR THERAPY

Similarly to metals, gems and stones and also colors contain energy vibrations with healing properties. The healing energy of gems and stones may be activated in the individual by wearing them as ornaments such as rings or necklaces; or by placing the gem stones in water overnight and drinking the water the next day. Gems may be purified by placing them in salt water for two days.

Gems give off as well as draw in energy through their negative and positive vibrations. They activate energy centers in the body and in this way help to develop sensitivity.

Following are lists of gems that are beneficial for individuals according to their birthdays as well as the descriptions of properties and uses of a number of well-known gems and stones.

Calendar of Birth Stones

January - garnet
February - amethyst
March - bloodstone
April - diamond
May - agate
June - pearl
July - ruby
August - sapphire
September - moonstone
October - opal
November - topaz
December - ruby

Uses of Gems

For healing - amethyst, bloodstone, pearl
To experience subtle effects of energy - diamond, lapis lazuli, ruby
To attract creativity - bloodstone, pearl
To develop psychic ability - lapis linquis
For receptivity - agate, beryl
To provide general protection - beryl, lapis linquis
For protection from cold - carbon steel
For protection against anger - pearl, opal

Agate. Smokey color. Agate will protect children against fear and help young children to walk earlier and to maintain their balance. This gem stimulates spiritual awakening. It helps to relieve *kapha* disorders. Agate contains the elements of Ether, Air and Fire. It should be worn around the neck on a gold necklace.

Amethyst. Purple, blue or violet. Amethyst contains the

elements Ether and Water. It gives the individual dignity, love, compassion and hope. This gem helps to control emotional temperament. It is good for *vata* and *pitta* imbalances. Amethyst should be worn around the neck on a gold necklace.

Beryl. Yellow, green or blue. Beryl contains Fire and Ether. It stimulates excess *pitta* but will relieve excess *vata* and *kapha*. This gem promotes intelligence, power, prestige and position in society and it also enhances the values of art and music. It should be worn around the neck on a silver necklace or worn on the left ring finger in a silver ring.

Bloodstone. This quartz stone contains small droplets of red color. It helps to check hemorrhage and is the best blood purifier. Bloodstone helps to promote the spiritual upbringing of children. It is good for liver and spleen disorders as well as anemia. This stone contains Fire and Water. It should be worn around the neck on a gold necklace near the heart.

Diamond. White, blue or red. The energy of this very precious gem stone brings subtle vibrations to the heart, brain and the deeper tissues. Red diamond has fiery energy that stimulates *pitta*. Blue diamond has cooling energy that calms *pitta* and stimulates *kapha*. Colorless diamond stimulates *vata*, calms *pitta* and stimulates *kapha*. In Ayurveda, the diamond is used as a heart tonic. For this treatment, the diamond should be placed in a glass of water overnight and the water drunk the next day.

The diamond is the best rejuvenating precious stone. It brings prosperity and is spiritually uplifting. It helps to create a close bond in relationships; thus, this gem is traditionally associated with marriage. It contains Ether, Air, Fire, Water and Earth. It should be worn on the right ring-finger in a gold ring. It should be noted that diamonds of low quality will have negative effects upon the body.

Garnet. A silicate material with a variety of colors such as red, brown, black, green, yellow and white. Red, yellow and brown have a heating effect and are beneficial for *vata* and *kapha* disorders. White and green are useful for *pitta*, for they are cooling. Red garnet has Fire and Earth elements; green has Fire and Air; white has Water. Garnet can be worn around the neck in a gold setting for *vata* and *kapha*; for *pitta*, a silver setting is preferable.

Lapis Lazuli. Blue, violet or green. This stone strengthens the eyes and is used to treat various eye problems. Lapis lazuli is a heavenly, sacred stone. It gives strength to the body, mind and consciousness and sensitizes the wearer to higher spiritual vibrations. It contains Fire, Ether and Water elements. Lapis lazuli is good for *vata* and *kapha*. It should be worn around the neck on a gold necklace.

Lapis Linquis. Blue. This stone has properties similar to those of lapis lazuli. It helps in meditation and brings good fortune.

Moonstone. Gray or white. This stone absorbs lunar energy as may be seen by its physical resemblance to the moon. Moonstone calms the mind and its cooling energy relieves *pitta*. It contains the elements of Water, Air and Ether. Moonstone is closely related to the human emotions and affects bodily water. If a person is suffering from emotional stress and experiences upsets at the new or full moon, he should wear a moonstone set in a silver ring on the right ring-finger. Moonstone will relieve disturbed *vata* as well as *pitta*; however, it will aggravate *kapha*.

Opal. Red, yellowish-red or orange-yellow. Opal aids a child's growth. It promotes benevolent feelings and friendship. It is the gem of God, of love and faith and of compassion, creativity and understanding in relationships. It contains Water, Fire and Ether. This stone is good for *vata* and *kapha* conditions. It should be worn on the right index-finger in a gold ring or around the neck on a gold necklace.

Pearl. White. This gem is an organic product from the mother-of-pearl (oyster). Pearl contains Water, Air and Earth. It contains calcium carbonate and it has a cooling effect and a calming, healing vibration. Pearl has anti-*pitta* properties. It also purifies the blood. In its purified ash form, pearl is used internally for stomach and inflammatory intestinal diseases. It may be employed in the treatment of hepatitis and gallstones. A person who is afflicted with biliary vomiting may be effectively treated with pearl-ash.

Pearl is a hemostatic. It is therefore used to treat disorders such as bleeding from the gums, vomiting with bleeding, bleeding through sputum or bleeding piles.

Pearl has strengthening qualities and promotes vigor and vitality. The electrical energy of the pearl may be harnessed by making pearl-water. Four or five small pearls should be placed in a glass of water and allowed to stand overnight. This water should be taken as a tonic the next day. It will alleviate a burning sensation of the eyes and also burning urine. Pearl-water also acts as a natural antacid and helps acute inflammatory conditions. Pearl should be worn on the right ring-finger in a silver ring.

Red coral. This gem stone which comes from the sea absorbs energy from the planet Mars. Red coral also contains calcium carbonate. Its action calms *pitta*. It is a blood purifier and helps one to control hate, anger and jealousy if worn either on the index or ring-finger of the right hand. It contains the elements Water, Earth and Fire.

Ruby. Red. This gem helps concentration and gives mental power. Ruby strengthens the heart. It contains the elements Fire, Air and Ether. *Pitta* is sensitive to this gem; however, it is good for excess *vata* and *kapha*. It should be worn on the left ring-finger in either a gold or silver ring.

Sapphire. Violet or purple color. Sapphire has a neutralizing effect on *vata*. It is used to counteract the negative effects of the planet Saturn, and helps in diseases like rheumatism, sciatica, neurological pain, epilepsy, hysteria and all *vata* disorders. It contains elements of Air and Ether. It should be worn around the neck in a gold setting.

Topaz. Straw-yellow, wine-yellow, greenish or reddish-blue. This gem promotes passion and relieves fear. Topaz gives strength and intelligence. It contains Fire, Ether and Air. It should be worn on the right index-finger in a gold ring or around the neck on a gold necklace.

COLOR

Ayurvedic treatments also employ the healing properties of certain colors. The seven basic natural colors, which are present in the rainbow, are related to the bodily tissues and the *tridosha.* Thus, the actions of the vibrations of these seven colors may be used to help establish the balance of the three humors.

If gelatinous paper of any of the seven colors is wrapped around a jar of water and placed in the sunlight for four hours, the water will become infused with the vibrations of the color. This water may then be taken internally with beneficial results. The following colors are used in Ayurvedic treatments:

Red. This color is related to the blood. It has a heating property, promotes the red color of the red blood cells and also stimulates the formation of red blood cells. Also, the color red creates heat in the body and stimulates circulation. It helps to maintain the color of the skin and gives energy to the nerve tissue and bone marrow. Red relieves aggravated *vata* and *kapha.* However, overexposure to this color may cause overabundance of *pitta* to collect in certain parts of the body, resulting in inflammation. Overexposure to red may cause conjunctivitis.

Orange. The color orange, like red, is warming and has healing energy. It helps the spiritual seeker to renounce the world. Yet it also gives energy and strength to the sex organs. Thus, orange should be used in conjunction with celibacy in order to transform sexual energy into Supreme Consciousness. One who is not celibate will be overstimulated sexually by the application of this color. Orange helps to relieve aggravated *vata* and *kapha.* It also

149

relieves congestion and maintains the luster of the skin. Over-exposure to orange may aggravate *pitta*.

Yellow. Energy rises to the crown *chakra* when one is exposed to the color yellow. This color stimulates understanding and intelligence. In spiritual terms, yellow is connected with the complete death of the ego. Overuse of this color causes excess accumulation of bile in the small intestine and may aggravate *pitta*. Yellow relieves excess *vata* and *kapha*.

Green. This color has a calming effect upon the mind and creates freshness. It helps to bring energy to the heart *chakra*. Green also soothes the emotions and brings happiness to the heart. It calms excess *vata* and *kapha* and aggravates *pitta*. Overuse of green stimulates the concentration of bile which may create stones in the gallbladder.

Yellow-green. This color has the properties both of yellow and green. It helps to relieve *vata* and *kapha* and it may aggravate *pitta*. It has a calming effect upon the mind.

Blue. This is the color of Pure Consciousness. It has a calming, cooling effect on the body and the mind. Blue relieves dispigmentation of the skin. It also helps to correct liver disorders and relieves aggravated *pitta*. Overuse of blue may cause aggravation of *vata* and *kapha* and may cause congestion.

Purple (violet). This is the color of Cosmic Consciousness which brings an awakening of awareness. It creates lightness in the body, and it opens the doors of perception. Purple relieves aggravated *pitta* and *kapha* but overuse may aggravate *vata*.

Conclusion

Ayurveda comprehensively illuminates the basic laws and principles governing life on earth. To understand Ayurveda is to understand the forces that engender our well-being as well as those that lie at the root of disease. This brief introduction has been an attempt to introduce the reader to this life-science in a concise and informative way. It represents only a fraction of the total wealth of Ayurvedic wisdom. However, the intention, in which the author hopes he has succeeded, has been to offer a basic appreciation of the vast potential and profound healing power of Ayurveda; and to supply practical knowledge applicable to the reader's daily life.

All the basic concepts of Ayurveda have been introduced here, yet the reader may still have unanswered questions about this science of life. In fact, this book may have raised more questions than it has answered. This may be unavoidable when one treats, in an introductory manner, an ancient system of wisdom that encompasses that vast horizon where human consciousness merges into Cosmic Consciousness.

The author hopes that he has communicated some of the basic truths of this profound science in a readily understandable manner. Only you, the reader, can judge if his effort has succeeded in its intention. Your comments regarding this book will be most welcome, for they will help considerably in producing the next projected text which is to be a more detailed treatment of this ancient life-science.

As the early chapters of this book began with the creation originating in Cosmic Consciousness and the formation of the five elements, it is natural to conclude at that point where these elements return again to their Source to continue the cosmic cycle of existence:

As death approaches the Earth element, the feeling of
the solidity and hardness of the body begins to melt.

The body seems very heavy. The boundaries of the body, its edge, are less solid. There is not so much a feeling of being "in" the body. One is less sensitive to impressions and feelings. One can no longer move the limbs at will. Peristalsis slows, the bowels no longer move without aid. The organs begin to shut down. As the Earth element continues to dissolve into the Water element, there is a feeling of flowingness, a liquidity as the solidity that has always intensified identification with the body begins to melt, a feeling of fluidity.

As the Water element begins to dissolve into the Fire element, the feeling of fluidity becomes more like a warm mist. The bodily fluids begin to slow, the mouth and eyes become dry, circulation slows, blood pressure drops. As the circulation begins to thicken and stop, blood settles in the lowest extremities. A feeling of lightness ensues.

As the Fire element dissolves into the Air element, feelings of warmth and cold dissipate, physical comfort and discomfort no longer have meaning. The body temperature drops until it reaches a stage where the body begins to cool and becomes pale. Digestion stops. A feeling of lightness, as of heat rising, becomes predominant. A feeling of dissolving into yet subtler and subtler boundarylessness.

As the Air element dissolves into Consciousness itself there is a feeling of edgelessness. The out breath having become longer than the in breath has dissolved into Space and there is no longer the experience of bodily form or function but just a sense of vast expanding airiness, a dissolving into pure being.*

---

*From *Who Dies* by Stephen Levine. Anchor Books, New York, 1982, pp. 269-270.

So the human nervous system returns to the Source of its being. Yet the ending of that cycle, as well as of this book, marks the beginning of the journey for you, the reader. It is now time to look into the living book, which is your body, mind and consciousness. True knowledge resides in that temple. In applying to your experience in that sanctuary the knowledge set forth here, you will find the only authentic and trustworthy demonstration of the truth of this text. The journey is long, but we will always return to the place whence we began.

APPENDIX A
Food Antidotes*

Food	Negative Effects	Antidotes
DAIRY PRODUCTS		
Cheese	Increases congestion and mucus; aggravates *pitta* and *kapha*	black pepper, chili peppers or cayenne
Eggs	Increases *pitta*; if taken raw, will increase *kapha*	parsley, cilantro, turmeric and onions
Ice Cream	Increases mucus, causes congestion	clove or cardamom
Sour cream	Increases mucus, causes congestion	coriander and cardamom
Yogurt	Increases mucus, causes congestion	cumin or ginger
FISH AND MEAT		
Fish	Increases *pitta*	coconut, lime, and lemon
Red meat	Heavy to digest	cayenne, cloves, or chili peppers
GRAINS		
Oats	Increase *kapha* and fat	turmeric, mustard seed or cumin
Rice	Increase *kapha* and fat	clove or peppercorn
Wheat	Increase *kapha* and fat	ginger
VEGETABLES		
Legumes	Produce gas and distention	garlic, cloves, black pepper, cayenne, ginger, rock salt or chili peppers

*Food antidotes should be used in preparation or while eating these foods.

Cabbage	Produces gas	cook in sunflower oil with turmeric and mustard seed
Garlic	Increases *pitta*	grated coconut and lemon
Green Salad	Produces gas	olive oil with lemon juice
Onion	Produces gas	cooked: or salt, lemon, yogurt and mustard seed
Potato	Produces gas	ghee with peppercorn
Tomato	Increases *kapha*	lime or cumin

FRUITS

Avocado	Increases *kapha*	turmeric, lemon, garlic and black pepper
Banana	Increases *pitta* and *kapha*	cardamom
Dry fruits	Creates dryness; may aggravate *vata*	soak in water
Mango	Produces diarrhea	ghee with cardamom
Melon	Causes water retention	grated coconut with coriander
Watermelon	Causes water retention	Salt with chili peppers

NUTS AND SEEDS

Nuts	Produce gas and increase *pitta*	soak overnight and cook with sesame oil and chili peppers
Peanut Butter	Heavy; has a sticking property; increases *pitta*; creates headache	ginger or roasted cumin powder
Seeds	May aggravate *pitta*	soak and bake to make lighter

155

MISCELLANEOUS

Alcohol	Stimulant; depressant effect	Chew ¼ teaspoon cumin seeds or 1-2 cardamom seeds
Black tea	Stimulant; depressant effect	ginger
Caffeine	Stimulant; has after-effect of depression	nutmeg powder with cardamom
Chocolate	Stimulant; also acts to depress the system	cardamom or cumin
Coffee	Stimulant; depresses the system	nutmeg powder with cardamom
Popcorn	Produces dryness and gas	add ghee
Sweets	Increase congestion	dry ginger powder
Tobacco	Aggravates *pitta* and stimulates *vata*	gotu kola, calamus root or celery seeds

APPENDIX B
First Aid Treatments

Acne: Apply a turmeric and sandalwood powder paste externally using half a teaspoonful of each and adding sufficient water to make a paste. One may also take a half cupful of aloe vera juice internally two times per day until the acne clears.

Asthma: Licorice and ginger tea is recommended. Use half a teaspoonful of the combined herbs in one cupful of water. Another remedy for internal use is one-fourth cupful of onion juice with one teaspoonful of honey and one-eighth teaspoonful of black pepper. This relieves the congestion and cough and alleviates breathlessness.

Backache: Apply ginger paste and then eucalyptus oil to the affected area.

Bad Breath: Cleanse the mouth with licorice powder and eat fennel seeds. One may also take one-half cupful of aloe vera juice twice a day until freshness is restored to the breath.

Bleeding (external): Apply ice or a sandalwood paste. The black ash of a burned cotton ball may also be applied to the site of external bleeding.

Bleeding (internal): Drink warm milk to which one-half teaspoonful of saffron and turmeric powder have been added.

Boils: To bring a skin boil to a head, apply cooked onions as a poultice or apply a paste of ginger powder and turmeric (one-half teaspoonful of each) directly to the boil.

Burns: Make a paste of fresh gel of aloe vera with a pinch of turmeric powder. *Ghee* or coconut oil also may be used.

Cold: Boil one teaspoonful of ginger powder in one quart of water and inhale the steam. Eucalyptus leaves boiled in the same way are also excellent for the relief of colds. Eucalyptus oil applied to the sides of the nose will help to relieve congestion. Calamus root powder may also be used as a snuff: inhale a pinch in each nostril.

Constipation: Take senna leaf tea (one teaspoonful to one cup of water), or take one teaspoonful of *ghee* in a glass of hot milk at bedtime. Another remedy is one glass of water boiled with one tablespoonful of flax seed to be drunk at bedtime.

Cough: Gargle one glass of warm water to which a pinch of salt and two pinches of turmeric powder have been added. Also suck a whole clove with a piece of rock candy. If a cough brings up mucus, take one-half teaspoonful of ginger powder, one pinch of clove and one pinch of cinnamon powder in one cupful of boiled water as a tea.

Diarrhea: Blend together equal parts of yogurt and water and add some fresh ginger (about one-eighth teaspoonful); or drink black coffee mixed with fresh lemon juice. Another remedy is gruel made with one to two teaspoonsful of poppy seeds in one cup of water. Boil this mixture, add a pinch of nutmeg, blend and eat.

Earache: Place three drops of garlic oil in the ear; or use a mixture of one teaspoonful of onion juice with one-half teaspoonful of honey and introduce five to ten drops into the ear.

Ears (ringing): Put three drops of clove oil into the ear. (See recipe section for clove oil — Appendix C.)

Exhaustion (heat): Drink one glassful of coconut water or grape juice. Or cook three dates with eight ounces of water, blend and drink.

Eyes (burning): Apply castor oil to the soles of the feet. Or introduce three drops of pure rose water into the affected eye. Fresh aloe vera gel may also be used in the eye.

Gas (abdominal): Mix one pinch of baking soda with one cupful of water and the juice of one-half lemon and drink.

Gums (bleeding): Drink the juice of one-half lemon squeezed into one cupful of water. Or massage the gums with coconut oil.

Headache: For general relief of headaches, a paste of one-half teaspoonful of ginger powder, mixed with water and heated, is applied to the forehead. A burning sensation may possibly occur, but it will not be harmful.

Another method for relief is the observation of breath. Notice if one nostril has a more forceful discharge of air. If it does, close that nostril and breathe through the other until headache subsides.

The following can be useful for relief of specific types of headaches. Sinus headaches relate to *kapha* and can be relieved by applying a ginger paste to the forehead and sinuses. Temporal headaches indicate an excess of *pitta* in the stomach. They can be relieved by drinking a tea of cumin and coriander seeds, one half teaspoonful of each in one cup of hot water. At the same time, apply a sandalwood paste to the temples. Occipital headaches indicate toxins in the colon. Take one teaspoonful of flaxseed at bedtime with a glass of warm milk. At the same time, apply a ginger paste behind the ears (mastoid processes).

Headaches may be due to a change in energy or to repressed emotions in the deep connective tissue.

Hemorrhoids: Drink one-half cupful of aloe vera juice three times a day until hemorrhoids disappear.

Hiccups: Take two parts honey with one part castor oil. Also do *pranayama.* (See Chapter XII — Breathing and Meditation.)

Indigestion: Eat one clove of minced garlic with a pinch of salt and a pinch of baking soda. Or take one-fourth cupful of onion juice with one-half teaspoonful of honey and one-half teaspoonful of black pepper.

Menstrual Cramps: Take one tablespoonful of aloe vera gel with two pinches of black pepper orally three times a day until cramps disappear.

Muscle Strain (upper body): An enema of one cupful of calamus oil may be injected into the rectum. Retain for thirty minutes. For general muscle strain, apply warm ginger paste with turmeric (one teaspoonful of ginger with one-half teaspoonful of turmeric) to the affected area twice a day.

Overeating: Overeating is a nervous habit that destroys the intelligence of the body. Eat light food like millet, tapioca or rye. These substances will not increase weight even if taken to excess. If you have already erred, roast one teaspoonful each of fennel seeds and coriander seeds with one pinch of salt and eat. You also may drink a cupful of warm water to which has been added the juice of one-half lemon and a pinch of baking soda.

Pain (external): Apply a ginger compress. To prepare a ginger compress, combine two teaspoonsful of ginger powder with one teaspoonful of turmeric powder and add enough water to make a paste. Warm the paste and spread it evenly on a piece of gauze or cotton cloth. Then place the cloth on the affected area and apply a bandage over it. Keep it on over night.

Poison Bites and Stings: Drink cilantro juice or apply a sandalwood paste to the affected area.

Poison (general): Take one-half teaspoonful of *ghee* or one-half teaspoonful of licorice powder.

Rash: Apply the pulp of cilantro leaf to the affected area or drink coriander tea (one teaspoonful of coriander seeds to one cupful of water).

Shock (fainting): Inhale fresh, broken onion, or inhale calamus root powder.

Sinus Congestion: Apply ginger paste to the affected area or inhale one pinch of calamus root powder.

Sleep (lack of): Drink a tea made with one-fourth teaspoonful of nutmeg powder to one cupful of water. Gently massage the soles of the feet with sesame oil; or rub the scalp with the oil; or introduce five to ten drops of warmed oil into each ear. Drink one cupful of hot cow's milk with rock candy or honey. Camomile tea is also excellent for inducing sleep (one tablespoonful of camomile in one cupful of water).

Sleep (excess): Drink coffee, gotu kola tea or calamus root tea at bedtime. Eat early in the evening and eat less.

Sore Throat: Gargle with hot water mixed with one-fourth teaspoonful of turmeric powder and a pinch of salt.

Swelling: Drink barley water: four parts of water boiled with one part of barley, then strain. Coriander tea also is beneficial. For external swelling, apply two parts of turmeric powder mixed with one part salt to the affected area. Drink gotu kola tea: one tablespoonful to one cup of water.

Toothache: Apply three drops of clove oil to the affected tooth.

APPENDIX C
Recipes

Almond Drink: Soak ten almonds overnight in water. In the morning remove the skins. Place almonds in a blender with one cup of warm milk. Add a pinchful each of cardamom powder and black pepper freshly ground from peppercorn, and one teaspoonful of honey. Blend for five minutes on high speed and drink. This drink helps to improve energy and *ojas*.

Buttermilk (lassi): Heat one quart of milk just to the boiling point. Let it simmer and squeeze a little lemon juice into it. Then add one tablespoonful of yogurt culture. Cover the milk and keep it in a warm, dark place over night. It will have become fresh yogurt by next morning. Add the yogurt to an equal amount of water and mix it in a blender. Maple syrup may be added as a sweetener.

Calamus Root Ghee: First prepare a calamus root decoction by taking one part of calamus root powder and adding to it eight parts of water. Boil this mixture until one-fourth of the water remains. Take one part of this decoction and add to it an equal part of *ghee* (see *ghee* recipe). To this mixture, add an equal part of water and boil until the water evaporates. What remains is calamus root *ghee*.

Clove Oil: Boil five whole cloves in one tablespoonful of sesame oil and leave the cloves in the oil. The oil should be warm when applied.

Garlic Oil: Crush two cloves of garlic and add to one tablespoonful of sesame oil. Boil. Leaving the garlic in the oil, apply the warm mixture.

Ghee: Heat one pound of unsalted butter on a medium fire. After butter melts, heat for about twelve minutes. As it boils, froth will rise to the surface. (Do not remove this foam for it contains medicinal properties.) Turn fire to low. The butter will turn a golden yellow color and will smell rather like popcorn. When a drop or two of water placed in the *ghee* produces a crackling sound, the *ghee* is ready. Let cool. Pour it through a strainer into a container. *Ghee* may be stored without refrigeration.

Licorice Ghee: First prepare a licorice decoction by taking one part of licorice powder and adding eight parts of water. Boil the liquid until one-fourth remains. Take one part of this decoction and add to it an equal part of *ghee* (see *ghee* recipe). Then add an equal part of water and boil until all the water evaporates. What remains is licorice *ghee*.

Yogi Tea: Mix the following ingredients together: two teaspoonsful of fresh grated ginger, four whole cardamom seeds, eight whole cloves, a whole cinnamon stick and eight cups of water. Boil until one-half the liquid remains. Add one ounce of cow's milk after the mixture has cooled and drink.

Glossary

Acne: An inflammatory eruption occurring usually on the face, neck, shoulders and upper back.

Afferent Nerves: Sensory nerve impulses which carry sensations to the brain

Allergy: A hypersensitive reaction to substances in the individual's environment

Allopathy: A system of medicine (Western medicine) which treats disease and injury with active interventions, e.g., medical and surgical treatment to bring about opposite effects from those produced by the disease or injury

Anabolism: The constructive or building-up process of the body (aspect of metabolism)

Analgesic: A substance that relieves pain

Anemia: A below-normal level in the number of red blood cells

Aromatic: Substances with a fragrant smell and a pungent, spicy taste which stimulate the gastrointestinal tract

Arthritis: An inflammatory condition of the joints, characterized by pain and swelling

Ascites: An excessive accumulation of fluid in the abdominal cavity

Asthma: A respiratory disorder in which there is breathlessness, wheezing and cough (dry or with expectoration)

Atrophy: A wasting or diminution of size or physiological activity of a part of the body, owing to disease or other influences

Attributes: The inherent qualities or properties of a substance

Auscultation: The act of listening for sounds within the body

Bile: A bitter fluid secreted by the liver which flows into the small intestine; stored in the gallbladder, it helps to metabolize fat

Bronchitis: Inflammation of the bronchials (in lungs)

Bursitis: Inflammation of the connective tissue structure surrounding a joint

Carminative: A substance that relieves gas

Catabolism: The destructive or breaking-down process in the body; aspect of metabolism (see Anabolism)

Cervicitis: Inflammation of the cervix which is the neck of the uterus

Chakra: Energy centers in the body that are responsible for the different levels of consciousness; they correspond physiologically to the nerve plexus centers

Charak: Great Ayurvedic physician who wrote one of the classic texts of Ayurveda: *Charak Samita*

Cholesterol: A fatty substance in crystalized form found in all animal fats, oils, milk, egg yolks, bile, blood, brain tissue, liver, kidney and adrenal glands.

Colitis: A chronic disease characterized by the excessive secretion of mucus in the large intestine and marked by constipation or diarrhea and the passage of mucus and membranous shreds in the feces

Compress: A pad of folded linen applied so as to create pressure upon exterior parts of the body

Conjunctivitis: An inflammation of the membrane that lines the eyelids

Cosmic energy: The all-pervading energy in the universe

Dermatitis: An inflammatory condition of the skin, characterized by redness, pain and itching

Diabetes: A clinical condition characterized by the excessive excretion of urine and increased blood-sugar level.

Dispigmentation: The loss of color of the skin

Distention: Bloating from internal pressure

Diuretic: A substance that increases the secretion of urine

Eczema: Acute or chronic skin inflammation

Edema: A condition in which the body tissues retain an excessive amount of fluid resulting in swelling

Efferent Nerves: Sensory nerve impulses which carry sensations away from the brain.

Electrolyte: An element or compound that, when melted or dissolved in water or other solvent, dissociates into ions to conduct an electric current

Emetic: Medicine that produces vomiting

Endocrine Glands: Glands whose function it is to secrete into the blood or lymph a substance that has a specific effect on organs or other parts of the body

Enteritis: An inflammation of the intestines usually the small intestine

Epilepsy: A group of neurological disorders characterized by recurrent episodes of convulsive seizures, sensory disturbances abnormal behavior, loss of consciousness, or all of these

Expectorant: A substance that promotes the ejection of mucus or other substances from the lungs, bronchi and trachea

Flora: Healthful bacteria which are present in various parts of the body, particularly the digestive tract

Fomentation: Treatment by warm and moist application

Gastrointestinal Tract: The organs from the mouth to the anus which are involved with ingestion, digestion, absorption and elimination

Gonorrhea: A common venereal disease most often affecting the genitourinary tract

Gout: Metabolic disease marked by acute arthritis and inflammation of the joints

Hemorrhoids: Enlarged veins in the lower rectum or anus owing to congestion

Hemoptysis: Coughing up of blood from the respiratory tract

Hemostatic: A substance that checks the flow of blood

Hives: Eruptions of very itchy skin caused by an allergic substance or food

Infusion: The steeping of a substance in water to obtain its proximate principles

Jaundice: A condition characterized by yellowness of the skin

Karma: Any action

Leucoderma: Localized loss of skin pigment

Leukorrhea: A condition that causes a whitish, viscid discharge from the vagina and uterine cavity

Lymphadenitis: Inflammatory condition of the lymph nodes

Macrocosm: The universe itself; a system regarded as an entity containing subsystems

Malabsorption syndrome: A condition in which there is no proper digestion, absorption and assimilation of food in the gastro-intestinal tract

Metabolism: The sum of all the biophysical and chemical processes through which living organisms function and maintain life. Also the transformation of substances (such as ingested food) by which energy is made available for the use of the organism

Microcosm: A diminutive representative world; a system more or less analogous to a much larger system

Palpation: The act of feeling with the hand; the application of the fingers ,with light pressure to the surface of the body for the purpose of determining the consistancy of the parts beneath

Parkinsonism: A neurologic disorder characterized by tremors, muscle rigidity and slow movements

Pathogenesis: Origination and development of a disease

Peristalsis: Rhythmic contraction of smooth muscle that forces food through the digestive tract

Percussion: The act of striking a bodily part with short, sharp blows as a diagnostic aid that reveals the condition of that area of the body

Pharyngitis: Inflammation of the throat

Physiognomy: The study of facial features

Poultice: A soft, moist substance applied hot to the surface of the body for the purpose of supplying heat and moisture

Prana: It is vital energy (life-energy) which activates the body and mind. *Prana* is responsible for the higher cerebral functions, and the motor and sensory activities. The *prana* located in the head is the vital *prana*, while *prana* which is present in the cosmic air is nutrient *prana*. There is a constant exchange of energy between vital *prana* and nutrient *prana* through respiration. During inspiration, the nutrient *prana* enters the system and nourishes the vital *prana*. During expiration, subtle waste products are expelled.

Psoriasis: A common genetically-determined skin inflammation

Psychosomatic: Pertaining to the mind-body relationship; having bodily symptoms of a psychic, emotional or mental origin

Ptosis: An abnormal condition of one or both upper eyelids in which the eyelid droops

Rheumatism: Any of a large number of inflammatory conditions of the joints, ligaments or muscles, characterized by pain or limitation of movement

Rhinitis: Inflammation of the mucus membrane of the nose

Samadhi: A state of equilibrium; supreme joy and bliss

Scabies: A contagious skin disease characterized by itching and peeling of the skin

Sciatica: Inflammation of the sciatic nerve characterized by lower back pain which radiates down the leg

Sinus: A cavity within a bone

Spondylosis: A condition of the spine characterized by fixation or stiffness of a vertebral joint

Syphilis: A venereal infection transmitted through sexual contact

Tridosha: The three bodily organizations — vata (air), pitta (fire) and kapha (water) — which govern the psychosomatic activity of daily living

Unctuous: Having the nature, characteristic or quality of an ointment

Urticaria: A blood reaction of the skin, marked by the transient appearance of smooth, slightly-elevated patches which are redder or paler than the surrounding skin. This condition often is attended by severe itching.

Bibliography

Charak Samhita. Varanasi, India: Chowkhamba Sanskrit Series, 1977.

Kudatarakar, Dr. M.N. *Vikriti Vijnyana*. India: Dhanvantari Prakashan, 1959.

Madhav Nidan. Varansi, India: Chowkhamba Sanskrit Series, 1963.

Pathak, Dr. R.R. *Therapeutic Guide to Ayurvedic Medicine*. Nagpur, India: Baidyanath, 1970.

Sharma, D.P., and Shastri, S.K. (eds.) *Basic Principles of Ayurveda*. Patna, India: Baidyanath Ayurveda Bhavan Ltd., 1978.

Sushrut Samhita. Varansi, India: Chowkhamba Sanskrit Series, 1963.

Udupa, K.N., and Singh, R.H. *Science and Philosophy of Indian Medicine*. Nagpur, India: Baidyanath, 1978.

Index

Abdominal pain, 134, 135, 139
Acidity, 38, 39, 42, 75, 131
Acne, 73, 78, 79, 107, 157
Activity level, 32, 34, 104
Adrenals, 114
Agate, 145
Ages, 107-108
Agni:
  Attributes, 50-51
  Dhatu-agni, 45, 111
  Diet & foods, 81, 85, 135
  Disorders, 40, 41, 64
  Fasting, 86
  Functions, 39, 45, 111
  Health, 37
  Herbs, 86, 131, 132, 133,
   136, 138, 140
  Prana, 109
  Treatment, 73, 79, 85
  Vitamins, 87
Ahamkar, 16
Ahara rasa, 45
Alcohol, 42
Alfalfa, 130
Allergies, 41, 70, 79
Almond Drink, 162
Aloe vera, 130, 157, 159
Ama, 39, 40
Amethyst, 145, 146
Anabolism, 31
Anemia, 59, 64, 65, 68, 78,
 130, 136, 143, 144, 146
Anger, 33, 40, 70, 103, 114,
 115, 145
Antacid, 131, 148
Antibacterial, 141
Antibiotics, 20
Antihistamines, 41
Antiseptic, 133
Anus, 25, 103
Anxiety, 32, 40, 62, 67
Appetite, 32, 33, 104, 136,
 139, 140
Appetizer, 133, 135, 136
Apple juice, 86
Aromatic, 132, 133, 134, 136,
 139, 141
Art, 146
Artav, 45
Arthritis, 38, 68, 75, 86, 108,
 130, 132, 141
Asafoetida, 130
Ascites, 44, 73
Asparagus root, 79
Asthi, 45
Asthma, 70, 107, 113, 115,
 116, 132, 135, 138, 140, 141,
 144, 157
Astral, 36, 142
Astrology, 107
Attributes, *see* Gunas
Aum, 16, 21, 126

Back pain, 38, 75, 115, 132, 157
Bacteria, 20, 39
Bad breath, 25, 42, 102, 132
Baking soda, 131, 159, 160
Barley water, 161
Basti, see Enema
Bathing, 100, 101, 137
Beans, 131
Beryl, 145, 146
Bhutas, see Elements
Bile, 38, 40, 42, 59, 70, 107,
 149, 150
Black pepper, 79, 86, 130, 140,
 157, 159
Bladder, 59
Bleeding, 73, 148, 157
Blood, 40, 78, 107, 136, 149
 see also Rakta
Blood clots, 133
Blood-letting, 78-79, 112
Blood pressure, 42, 113, 115
Blood purification, 79, 112, 130,
 134, 137, 141, 146
Bloodstone, 145, 146
Blood vessels, 40, 45
Blue, 150
Body odor, 102
Body temperature, 44
Boil, 139, 157
Bones, 32, 33, 45, 64, 78, 110,
 114, 143, *see also* Asthi
Brahma, 16
Brain, 65, 75, 131, 137,
 139, 146
Breakfast, 100, 101, 104
Breathing, 70, 76, 78, 101,
 108, 132, 157
Breathing exercises,
 see Pranayama
Bronchitis, 38, 70, 105, 116,
 138
Bruise, 141
Burdock, 78
Burns, 130, 157
Buttermilk, 101, 134, 162

Calamus, 70, 79, 131-132, 136,
 159, 160, 161, 162
Calamus oil, 75, 128, 132, 158
Calcium, 65, 67, 109
Calming, 102, 112, 128, 137,
 147, 149, 150
Camomile, 160
Carbon steel, 145
Cardamom, 132, 133, 163
Carminative, 136, 138
Cashews, 103
Castor oil, 132, 159
Catabolism, 31
Cayenne, 86, 133
Celibacy, 110, 112, 135,
 139, 149

Cervicitis, 130
Chakras, 110, 149
Charak, 48, 89
Cheese, 133
Cholesterol, 136, 140
Cilantro, 134, 160
Cinnamon, 133, 158, 163
Circulation, 102, 128, 131, 132,
 137, 149
Cleansing, 70-79, 111, 113, 133
 see also Pancha Karma
Climate, 85
Cloves, 133, 158, 161, 162, 163
Coconut, 158
Coconut oil, 159
Coffee, 42, 158, 161
Cold, 41, 70, 75, 86, 105, 107,
 130, 131, 133, 134, 136, 137,
 138, 158
Cold drinks, 85, 102, 125
Colitis, 107, 115, 130, 136
Colon, *see* Large Intestine
Color therapy, 144, 149-150
Congestion, 41, 70, 75, 105,
 130, 132, 133, 134, 135, 136,
 137, 138, 141, 149, 150, 157
Conjunctivitis, 130, 149
Consciousness, 19, 25, 105,
 110, 112, 126, 131, 137
Constipation, 25, 42, 73, 75,
 86, 102, 115, 132, 135,
 138, 140, 158
Constitution, 26-36, 34-35, 36,
 38, 56, 64, 80, 85, 87, 100,
 101, 114, 128
Convulsions, 75, 139
 see also Epilepsy
Copper, 102, 142-143
Coral, red, 148
Coriander, 134, 160, 161
Corn oil, 128
Cosmic Consciousness, 15, 21,
 22, 126, 137, 150
Cotton ash, 157
Cough, 41, 70, 105, 107, 130,
 132, 133, 134, 135, 136, 137,
 138, 140, 141, 157, 158
Creation, 17, 21
Cumin, 101, 134
Curry, 86, 140
Cuts, 130

Dandruff, 44
Dates, 158
Death, 110, 112, 151-153
Decongestant, 134, 137
Dehydration, 44, 64
Depression, 115
Dermatitis, 44, 73, 105, 134,
 140, 141
Deviated nasal septum, 76
Dhatus, 13, 44-47, 109, 110, 111
Diabetes, 44, 70, 110, 113,
 116, 138, 141, 144
Diagnosis, 43, 52-68
Diamond, 145, 146

Diarrhea, 42, 73, 105, 134, 139, 158
Diet, 73, 80-85, 101-102, 154-156
Digestion:
  Aids, 79, 85, 101-102, 130, 131, 133, 134, 135, 136, 138, 139, 140, 141, 160
  Disorders, 40, 64, 65, 70, 81, 115, 160
  Physiology, 32, 33, 39, 104, 111
Dinner, 100, 105
Disease, 37, 40, 41, 47, 52, 125
Distention, 42, 75, 135, 139, 140
Diuretic, 134
Dizziness, 139
Dreams, 105
Dysentery, 134

Ears, 23, 76, 103, 131, 135, 158
Eating routine, 81, 85, 101, 104-105
Eczema, 78
Edema, 42, 64, 70, 78, 85, 143
Ego, 16, 149
Electrolytes, 42
Elements, five basic, 13, 16, 21-26, 51, 57, 88, 110, 151-152
Emaciation, 31, 40, 107, 108, 144
Emetic, 131, 138
Emotions, 30, 38, 39, 40-41, 62, 69, 70, 76, 86, 103, 105, 109, 112, 146, 147, 149
Emphysema, 116
Enema, 73-75, 111, 112, 159
Energy, 22, 103, 104, 137
Environment, 37, 105
Enzymes, 39, 81, 85, 111, 144
Epilepsy, 70, 107, 131, 140, 143
  see also Convulsions
Eucalyptus, 157, 158
Exercise, 79, 100
Exhaustion, heat, 158
Expectorant, 130, 131, 134, 138
Eye diagnosis, 67-68
Eyelids, 62
Eyes, 23, 32, 33, 68, 76, 78, 100, 102, 103, 105, 136, 137, 146, 148, 159

Facial diagnosis, 62-64
Fainting, 139, 160
Fasting, 79, 85-87, 101, 102
Fat, 45, 122, 125, 137, 142
  see also Meda
Fatigue, 32
Fear, 32, 40, 64, 67, 70, 103, 110, 114, 145, 148
Feces, 32, 33, 34, 41-42, 135
Feet, 23, 32, 33, 44, 102, 105
Female energy, 15, 16, 48, 101, 114, 126
Fennel, 157, 160

Fever, 42, 73, 75, 86, 102, 136, 139, 144
First aid, 157-161
Flax seeds, 134, 158
Flora, 39, 40, 44, 141
Folic acid, 64
Food antidotes, 154-156
Fresh air, 79
Fungus, 44

Gallbladder, 38, 40, 59, 130, 138, 144
Gallstones, 147, 150
Garlic, 135, 136, 139, 158, 159, 162
Garnet, 145, 146-147
Gas, 38, 40, 42, 70, 88, 131, 132, 134, 135, 139, 140, 141, 159
Gastritis, 38, 138
Gems, 144-148
Genitals, 23
Germicide, 138
Ghee, 73, 76, 101, 110, 135-136, 138, 140, 158, 160, 162, 163
Ginger, 79, 86, 101, 102, 132, 133, 136, 157, 158, 159, 160, 163
Gold, 131, 143
Gonorrhea, 143, 144
Gotu kola, 136, 137, 161
Gout, 75, 78, 132
Grape juice, 86, 158
Greed, 34, 70, 103
Green, 150
Growth, 147
Gums, 101, 135, 148, 159
Gunas, 16, 36, 48-51, 105, 123

Hair, 32, 33, 102
Hands, 23, 32, 33, 44, 101
Headache, 42, 75, 115, 116, 131, 135, 136, 159
Health, 18, 37, 52, 80, 111
Heart, 40, 59, 64, 65, 67, 70, 75, 103, 110, 125, 132, 139, 140, 142, 143, 144, 146, 148, 150
Heartburn, 144
Height, 32
Hemorrhage, 146
Hemorrhoids, 115, 140, 141, 148, 159
Hepatitis, 147
Herbs, 129-141
Herpes, 64, 130
Hiccups, 159
Hives, 38, 105, 107, 131, 134, 140
Hoarseness, 75
Honey, 89, 132, 137, 157, 158, 159, 160
Hormones, 110, 113

Humors, see Tridosha
Hypertension, see Blood Pressure
Hysteria, 143

Immunity, 37, 38, 39, 40, 41, 45, 78, 102, 110, 111
Incompatible foods, 40, 81
Infections, 131
Inflammation, 38, 130, 132, 138, 141, 148, 149
Insomnia, 115, 139
Instincts, 18
Intelligence, 33, 39, 109, 110, 131, 135, 137, 143, 144, 146, 148, 149
Intestines, 70, 116, 136, 138, 144, 137
Iron, 64, 65, 68, 109, 143

Jaundice, 42, 64, 65, 73
Joints, 68, 103, 110, 135, 136, 138-139, 140

Kapha:
  Ages, 31, 107
  Attributes, 48-49, 50-51, 105, 123
  Colors, 149, 150
  Constitution, 26, 33-35
  Diagnosis, 43, 54, 56, 60, 64, 65, 66, 67, 68
  Diet and foods, 41, 81, 82-84, 90-99, 104, 107, 135, 136, 137, 140, 154, 155
  Disorders, 38, 64, 76, 107, 110
  Emotions, 38-39, 41, 70, 103
  Fasting, 86
  Functions, 26, 28, 30, 109
  Gems, 145, 146, 147, 148
  Herbs, 130, 131, 132, 133, 134, 136, 139
  Metals, 142, 144
  Pranayama, 114, 122
  Seasons, 105, 106
  Seats of, 27, 30
  Sleep, 101, 102
  Tastes, 88, 90-99B
  Time, 104, 106
  Treatment, 70, 71-72, 76-77, 112, 128, 140
  Yoga, 114, 115-116, 123-124
Karma, 112
Kidneys, 44, 59, 62, 67, 70, 71, 100, 137, 142
Kidney stones, 75

Lapis lazuli, 145, 147
Lapis linquis, 145, 147
Large intestine, 38, 39, 40, 41, 42, 44, 56, 58, 62, 64, 73, 86, 100, 102, 112, 130, 133, 141
Lassi, see Buttermilk

173

Laxative, 42, 79, 130, 131, 132, 133, 134, 141
see also Purgatives
Lead, 142, 143
Left side, 101
Lemon, 89, 131, 158, 159, 160
Lentils, 131, 133
Leucoderma, 78
Leukorrhea, 143
Licorice, 70, 136, 138, 157, 160, 163
Light sensitivity, 68
Lip diagnosis, 64, 65
Liver, 38, 40, 59, 62, 65, 68, 70, 78, 102, 107, 115, 130, 131, 139, 142, 143, 144, 146, 150
Longevity, 19, 39, 85, 109-112
Lunar energy, see Moon
Lunch, 100, 104
Lungs, 38, 58, 59, 65, 70, 125, 132, 143
Lymph, 70, 142, 143, 144

Mahad, 16
Mahesha, 16
Majja, 45
Malas, 37, 41-44, 111
Male energy, 15, 16, 48, 101, 114, 126
Mamsa, 45
Mantra, 125-128
Marijuana, 131
Marrow, 45, 143, 149
see also Majja
Mars, 107, 148
Massage, 100, 102, 128, 132
Masturbation, 103, 111
Matter, 21-22, 104, 142
Meat, 133
Meda, 45
Meditation, 100, 112, 114, 125-128, 147
Memory, 32, 108, 109, 132, 135, 137, 143
Menstrual disorders, 115, 130, 144, 160
Menstruation, 103, 107
Mental disorders, 32, 107, 114
Mercury (metal), 143-144
Mercury (planet), 107
Meridians, 56-57
Metabolism, 29, 39, 64, 111, 113
Metals, 141-144
Milk, cow's, 73, 102, 103, 107, 135, 139, 144, 157, 158, 160
Milk, mother's, 107, 110, 131
Millet, 160
Mind, 19, 105, 109, 112, 132, 149
Money, 32, 33, 34, 146
Moon, 101, 105, 107, 147
Moonstone, 145, 147
Mouth, 100, 102, 138, 140
Mucus, 70, 102, 107, 135, 137, 138, 158

Muscles, 32, 33, 45, 107, 128, 131, 132, 137, 138-139, 143, 160. see also Mamsa
Music, 146
Mustard, 138

Nadis, 125
Nails, 32, 33, 64-67, 103
Napping, 102
Nasal administration, 75-78, 112, 131, 132, 134, 140
Nasya, see Nasal Administration
Nausea, 134, 140
Neck, 75
Nerves, 45, 107, 143, 149
see also, Majja
Nervousness, 32, 64, 67, 103
Neuralgia, 38
Nose, 25, 32, 64, 75, 103, 136, 140
Numbness, 110
Nutmeg, 139, 158, 160
Nutrition, 42, 45, 46, 65, 111

Obesity, 102, 122, 143
Ojas, 109, 110, 111, 135, 162
Onion, 89, 139-140, 157, 158, 159, 160
Opal, 145, 147
Orange (color), 149-150
Orange juice, 79
Overeating, 85, 102, 160
Oxygenation, 109

Pain reliever, 130, 131, 132, 133, 134, 136, 138, 140, 141, 160
Palliation, 79
Pancha karma, 70-79, 111
Patanjali, 113
Paralysis, 38
Parasites, 41, 64, 103, 133, 140
Pearl, 145, 147-148
Pericardium, 59
Perspiration, 32, 33, 34, 41, 42, 44, 133, 136
Pharyngitis, 105
Pitta:
  Ages, 31, 108
  Attributes, 48, 50-51, 123
  Colors, 149, 150
  Constitution, 26, 32-33, 34-35
  Diagnosis, 43, 54, 56, 60, 64, 65, 66, 67, 68
  Diet and foods, 41, 42, 80, 81, 82-84, 90-99, 104, 135, 136, 137, 140, 154, 155
  Disorders, 38, 42, 64, 77, 78, 107
  Emotions, 38-39, 40, 41, 70, 103

Pitta, continued:
  Fasting, 86
  Functions, 26, 28, 30, 39, 44, 109
  Gems, 146, 147, 148
  Herbs, 130, 133, 134, 136, 138, 139, 140, 141
  Metals, 143, 144
  Pranayama, 114
  Seasons, 105, 106
  Seats, of, 27, 30
  Sleep, 101
  Tastes, 88, 90-99B
  Time, 104, 106
  Treatment, 72-73, 75, 77, 78, 112, 128
  Yoga, 114, 115-116, 123-124
Plasma, 45. see also Rasa
Poison, 160
Poison bites, 160
Pomegranate, 79, 86, 89
Poppy seeds, 158
Prabhav, 89
Prakruti, 16, 29
  see also Constitution
Prana, 56, 75, 109-110, 111, 125, 126, 142
Pranayama, 80, 100, 101, 110, 114, 122, 125, 126, 127, 159
Pregnancy, 110
Protein, 141
Psoriasis, 44
Psychedelics, 131
Pulse diagnosis, 52-59
Purgatives, 70, 72-73, 111, 112
  see also Laxatives
Purple, 150
Purusha, 16

Rajas, 16, 36, 135, 139
Rakta, 45, 60
Rakta moksha, see Blood Letting
Rasa (plasma), 45, 60
Rasa (taste) 88-89, 92-99B
Rash, 38, 70, 78, 79, 105, 131, 134, 143, 161
Recipes, 162-163
Red, 149
Red blood cells, 65, 143, 149
Rejuvenation, 19, 109, 111-112, 135, 143, 144, 146
Relaxant, 137, 139, 143
Repression, 40-41, 69
Reproductive tissues, 45
  see also Shukra and Artav
Rheumatism, 75, 115, 130, 132, 135
Rice, 101
Right side, 101
Rishis, 15, 21
Rock candy, 134, 158, 160
Rose water, 159
Routine, 100-103
Ruby, 145, 148
Running, 103, 122
Rye, 160

174

Saffron, 79, 157
Salivation, 138
Salt, 68, 70, 78, 101, 136, 140,
    141, 144, 158, 159, 160, 161
Samadhi, 126
Samkhya philosophy, 15, 17
Sandalwood, 79, 128, 157, 160
Sanskrit, 14, 125
Sapphire, 145, 148-149
Saturn, 107
Satva, 16, 36
Scabies, 78
Sciatica, 38, 75, 115, 130, 132
Seasons, 48, 81, 105, 106
Self-realization, 19, 36
Senna, 73, 158
Senses, 16, 23-25, 37, 110, 139
Sesame oil, 75, 101, 102, 128,
    139, 160, 162
Sexual disorders, 75, 107, 115,
    139
Sexual energy, 103, 135, 139,
    149
Sexual intercourse, 103, 111
Shakti, 15
Shavasan, 102
Shiva, 15, 144
Shock, 161
Shukra, 45, 110
Silver, 142, 144
Sinuses, 70, 75, 102, 116, 131,
    134, 136, 137, 161
Sinusitis, 38
Skin, 23, 32, 33, 38, 39, 44, 70,
    78, 128, 131, 134, 136, 141,
    143, 144, 149, 150
Skull, 65
Sleep, 32, 33, 34, 100, 101, 102
    104, 105, 137, 139, 161
Small intestine, 38, 39, 40, 59,
    62, 65, 112, 149
Smoking, 64
Speech, 23, 32
Spine, 62, 114
Spirituality, 110, 112, 135, 145,
    146, 147, 149
Spleen, 59, 62, 70, 78, 102,
    139, 142, 143, 144, 146
Stamina, 34, 86, 143, 144
Stimulant, 131, 132, 133, 136,
    141
Stomach, 38, 39, 40, 59, 62, 70,
    85, 105, 112, 130, 138, 147
Stomatitis, 115
Strength, 110, 144, 147, 148
Stress, 68, 112, 113, 137
Sugar, 68, 78, 103
Sulphur, 144
Sun, 101, 102, 104, 105, 107
Sunbathing, 79
Sunflower oil, 128
Sushruta, 13-14
Sweat, see Perspiration
Swelling, 140, 141, 143, 161
Syphilis, 143, 144

Talking, 103
Tamari, 89
Tamas, 16, 36
Tamatras, 16
Tantra, 18-19, 110
Tapioca, 160
Tastes, 32, 33, 34, 80, 81, 85,
    88-99B, 140
Tea, 42
Teeth, 100, 101, 135, 137, 138
Tejas, 109, 110, 111
Tendons, 31, 32, 33
Thirst, 79, 81
Throat, 100, 116, 136, 141, 161
Thyroid, 68, 115
Time, 104-108
Tin, 144
Tissues, see Dhatus
Tongue, 23, 40, 59-62, 88, 100
Tonic, 130, 141
Tonsillitis, 38, 70, 141
Toothache, 133, 135, 161
Topaz, 145, 149
Toxins, 62, 69, 78, 79, 81, 85,
    86, 101, 102, 103, 107, 113,
    130, 131, 132, 133, 136, 138
    see also Ama
Tremors, 108
Tridosha, 13, 26-31, 37, 38, 39,
    47, 49, 51, 52, 59, 69, 81,
    82, 89, 106, 111, 136, 148
    see also Kapha, Pitta and Vata
Tumor, 111
Turmeric, 79, 89, 130, 140, 141,
    157, 158, 159, 160, 161

Ulcers, 38, 107, 115, 130,
    136, 137, 138, 141
Upanishads, 18
Urges, 41, 102
Urine, 32, 33, 41-44, 134, 139,
    148

Vaginal discharges, 143
Vaginitis, 130
Vamana, see Vomiting Therapy
Varicose veins, 115
Vata:
    Ages, 31, 108
    Attributes, 48-49, 50-51, 123
    Colors, 149, 150
    Constitution, 26, 31-32, 34-35
    Diagnosis, 43, 54, 56, 60, 64,
        65, 66, 67, 68
    Diet and foods, 80, 81, 82-84,
        90-99, 104, 135, 136, 137,
        155
    Disorders, 31, 38, 64, 75, 77,
        103 108, 110
    Emotions, 38-39, 41, 70
    Fasting, 86
    Functions, 26, 28, 29-30, 109
    Gems, 146, 147, 148

Vata, continued:
    Herbs, 130, 132, 133, 136,
        139
    Metals, 144
    Pranayama, 114
    Seasons, 105, 106
    Seats of, 27, 30
    Sleep, 101
    Tastes, 88, 90-99B
    Time, 104, 106
    Treatment, 73, 74-77, 100,
        102, 112, 128
    Yoga, 114, 115-116, 123-124
Vedas, 18
Veins, 31, 32, 33
Venus, 107
Vipak, 88-89, 92-99B
Virechan, see Purgatives
Virya, 88-89, 92-99B
Vishnu, 16
Vitamins, 87
Vomiting, 73, 75, 134, 140,
    147, 148
Vomiting therapy, 70, 71-72,
    111, 112, 131, 138
    see also Emetic

Walking, 32, 101, 145
Waste products, 100, 101, 104
    see also Malas
Water, 22, 85, 87, 88, 100,
    102, 105, 107
Water retention, see Edema
Weakness, 78, 110, 139, 144
Weight, 33, 102, 143
Western medicine, 19-20, 87,
    129
Wheezing, 41, 70
Willpower, 32
Worms, see Parasites
Worry, 103
Wounds, 130, 136, 137, 138
Wrinkles, 62, 108, 115

Yellow, 150
Yellow dock, 141
Yellow-green, 150
Yoga, 18-19, 36, 80, 103, 112,
    113-124
Yogi tea, 163
Yogurt, 78, 158, 162

175

ABOUT THE AUTHOR

DR. VASANT LAD M.A.Sc., brings a wealth of classroom and practical experience to the United States. A native of India, he served for three years as Medical Director of the Ayurveda Hospital in Pune, India. He also held the position of Professor of Clinical Medicine at the Pune University College of Ayurvedic Medicine where he instructed for 15 years. Dr. Lad's academic and practical training included the study of allopathy (Western Medicine) and surgery as well as traditional Ayurveda. Beginning in 1979, he has traveled throughout the United States sharing his knowledge of Ayurveda, and in 1984, he returned to Albuquerque as Director of the Ayurvedic Institute.

Dr. Lad is also the author of AYURVEDA, THE SCIENCE OF SELF HEALING and many published articles on various aspects of Ayurveda. He presently directs the Ayurvedic Institute in Albuquerque and teaches the three semester Ayurvedic Studies Certificate Program. Dr. Lad also travels extensively in North America throughout the year, consulting privately and giving seminars on Ayurveda; history, theory, principles and practical applications.

THE AYURVEDIC INSTITUTE, ALBUQUERQUE, NM

Founded in 1984, the Ayurvedic Institute was established to promote an understanding of Ayurveda, probably the oldest system of total health (mental, physical and spiritual) known to man.
THE INSTITUTE offers certificate courses, seminars including Jyotisha and Sanskrit, a correspondence course in Ayurveda and membership which includes the quarterly journal "Ayurveda Today".
THE WELLNESS CENTER, incorporated within the Institute, offers consultations with Dr. Lad in person and over the phone, Pancha Karma and other Ayurvedic Treatments.
THE HERB DEPARTMENT, dispenses herbs and herbal compounds as well as Ayurvedic tinctures, oils and other products. Books pamphlets, audio and video tapes on Ayurveda are also available.

THE AYURVEDIC INSTITUTE
11311 Menaul NE
Albuquerque, NM 87112
(505) 291-9698

Yoga of Herbs
Complete Book of Ayurveda

The Yoga of Herbs
An Ayurvedic Guide to Herbal Medicine
Second Revised and Enlarged Edition

by Dr. Vasant Lad & Dr. David Frawley

For the first time, here is a detailed explanation and classification of herbs, using the ancient system of Ayurveda. More than 270 herbs are listed, with 108 herbs explained in detail. Included are many of the most commonly used western herbs with a profound Ayurvedic perspective. Important Chinese and special Ayurvedic herbs are introduced. Beautiful diagrams and charts, as well as detailed glossaries, appendices and index are included.

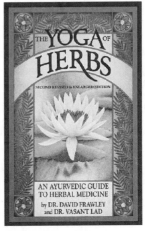

"Dr. Frawley and Dr. Lad have made a truly powerful contribution to alternative, natural health care by their creation of this important book. This book...will serve not only to make Ayurvedic medicine of greater practical value to Westerners but, in fact, ultimately advance the whole system of Western herbalism forward into greater effectiveness. I think anyone interested in herbs should closely study this book whether their interests lie in Western herbology, traditional Chinese herbology or in Ayurvedic medicine."

— Michael Tierra, Author, *The Way of Herbs*

Trade Paper   ISBN 978-0-9415-2424-7   288 pp   pb $15.95

Available at bookstores and natural food stores nationwide or order your copy directly by sending $15.95 plus $2.50 shipping/handling ($.75 s/h for each additional copy ordered at the same time) to:

Lotus Press, PO Box 325, Dept. AY, Twin Lakes, WI 53181 USA
toll free order line: 800 824 6396   office phone: 262 889 8561
office fax: 262 889 2461   email: lotuspress@lotuspress.com
web site: www.lotuspress.com

Lotus Press is the publisher of a wide range of books and software in the field of alternative health, including Ayurveda, Chinese medicine, herbology, aromatherapy, Reiki and energetic healing modalities. Request our free book catalog.

Ayurveda
La ciencia de curarse uno mismo
by Dr. Vasant Lad

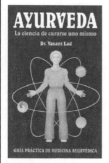

SPANISH EDITION
Este es el primer libro que explica con claridad los principios y aplicaciones prácticas de la Ayurveda, el sistema curativo más antiguo del mundo. El texto, bellamente ilustrado, trata, entre otros temas, lo siguiente historia y filosofía, principios básicos, técnicas de diagnóstico, tratamientos, uso medicinal de hierbas y especies y primeros anuxilios.

Se incluyen numerosas tablas y diagramas, que ayudan a comprender y aplicar mejor esta maravillosa ciencia de curar.

Trade Paper (English Edition)   ISBN 978-0-9149-5500-9   175 pp   pb $10.95

Trade Paper (Spanish Edition) ISBN 978-0-9409-8557-5   176 pp   pb $12.95

The Ayurvedic Cookbook
A Personalized Guide to Good Nutrition and Health
by Amadea Morningstar with Urmila Desai

The Ayurvedic Cookbook gives a fresh new perspective on this ancient art of self-healing. Over 250 taste-tested recipes are specifically designed to balance each constitution, with an emphasis on simplicity, ease and sound nutrition. Designed for the Western diner, recipes range from exotic Indian meals to old American favorites. Amadea Morningstar, M.A., a Western trained nutritionist, and Urmila Desai, a superb Indian cook, are both well-versed in a variety of healing traditions. *The Ayurvedic Cookbook* includes an in-depth discussion of Ayurvedic nutrition, tridoshic perspectives and ways to make dietary changes that last.

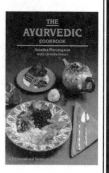

Trade Paper   ISBN 978-0-9149-5506-1   351 pp $17.95

Available at bookstores and natural food stores nationwide or order your copy directly by sending $17.95 plus $2.50 shipping/handling ($1.50 s/h for each additional copy ordered at the same time) to:

Lotus Press, P O Box 325, Twin Lakes, WI 53181 USA
toll free order line: 800 824 6396 office phone: 262 889 8561
office fax: 262 889 8591 email: lotuspress@lotuspress.com
web site: www.lotuspress.com